Advance Praise for *Bumpology* by Linda Geddes

"Finally! A book on pregnancy, birth, and babies that cuts through the myths, sidesteps preachy prescriptions, and turns to the evidence. *Bumpology* transforms common parental anxieties into fuel for a fascinating journey through the science of the bump."

—Hannah Devlin, science editor, *The Times* (London)

"[Geddes] combines scientific research with a light and humorous tone to answer burning questions."

—*The Bookseller*

"This book answers all the common pregnancy, birth, and newborn questions. . . . Thought-provoking and never boring, I loved it."

—*Mother & Baby*

"What a BRILLIANT book! The antidote to anecdote, a great survey of current evidence. Just what the midwife ordered!"

—Alice Roberts, professor of public engagement in science,
University of Birmingham

"Linda Geddes is not afraid to ask anyone about anything! From the stream of contradictory advice to pregnant women and new parents to those little moments of wonder, Geddes digs into all of them, looking for the evidence and exploring the science. In this book she shares what she's found, with the straightforward answers and easygoing humor that is so welcome in early parenthood. Don't get pregnant without it!"

—Tracey Brown, managing director, *Sense About Science*

LINDa GEDDES

Simon & Schuster Paperbacks
New York   London   Toronto   Sydney   New Delhi

BUMPology

The Myth-Busting Pregnancy Book
for Curious Parents-To-Be

Simon & Schuster
1230 Avenue of the Americas
New York, NY 10020

First Simon & Schuster paperback edition March 2014

SIMON & SCHUSTER and colophon are registered trademarks of Simon & Schuster, Inc.

For information about special discounts for bulk purchases, please contact Simon & Schuster Special Sales at 1-866-506-1949 or business@simonandschuster.com.

The Simon & Schuster Speakers Bureau can bring authors to your live event. For more information or to book an event contact the Simon & Schuster Speakers Bureau at 1-866-248-3049 or visit our website at www.simonspeakers.com.

Designed by Akasha Archer

Manufactured in the United States of America

10 9 8 7 6 5 4 3 2 1

Library of Congress Cataloging-in-Publication Data
Geddes, Linda.
Bumpology : the myth-busting pregnancy book for curious parents-to-be / Linda Geddes.
pages cm
1. Pregnancy—Popular works. 2. Childbirth—Popular works.
3. Infants—Care—Popular works. I. Title.
RG525.G39 2013
618.2—dc23
2013026987

ISBN 978-1-4516-8499-5
ISBN 978-1-4516-8577-0 (ebook)

To Matilda and Max

contents

TWO: BIrTH

Get a Move On

The Big Push

Ouch!

THREE: BABIES

Sleep

The White Stuff

Weaning

The Brown Stuff

Baby Brains

Language

The Next One

Foreword

As a newly pregnant woman, I was bursting with questions about my developing child. I remember having my twelve-week scan and spending the following weeks obsessing over what this jelly bean–shaped blob (which already showed signs of extraordinary wit and intelligence) was doing in there. Could it tell when I was in an airplane, in a swimming pool, or lying down to go to sleep? Could it taste the chicken jalfrezi I was eating at the local Indian restaurant, know that it was nighttime, or remember the sensation of that ill-advised Tilt-A-Whirl ride I took at the fairground?

I was also bemused by conflicting advice on eating, drinking, and exercise, much of which seemed to fly in the face of common sense. When I logged on to pregnancy forums, I realized that other women were asking similar questions, often falling back on anecdote and received wisdom, which provided unsatisfactory answers in general.

As a science journalist, I made it my job to indulge my curiosity and investigate the truth behind the old wives' tales, alarming newspaper headlines, and government guidelines. So *Bumpology* was born. What started as a fourteen-part blog for the *New Scientist* during the latter weeks of my first pregnancy developed into a two-and-a-half-year obsession with the science of bumps, birth, and newborn babies.

As our pregnancies developed, new and unexpected questions struck my pregnant friends and me, and as "B-day" approached and our thoughts (and worries) turned to the process of birth itself, I found myself asking even more.

The journey didn't stop there. Once my daughter, Matilda, was born, a whole new world of experiences and unresolved queries tugged at my curious mind. In the darkest hours of sleep deprivation, I wondered if babies could tell the difference between night and day and whether the personality traits that babies seem to be born with would follow them into later life; when my baby's diaper exploded, I considered the sterility of baby poop; and as my daughter grew more mobile and started to develop language, I contemplated just when and how qualities such as long-term memory and empathy develop.

As it turned out, many of the answers were already out there, buried in scientific journals or lodged in the brains of academics. It just took some digging to find them.

Shortly after starting to write this book, I discovered I was pregnant with my second child, Max. This time was a very different experience. The more I researched, the more I realized that much of what I had been told during my first pregnancy was not backed up by evidence, and in some cases—such as being told that if I requested epidural pain relief, I was more likely to need a C-section—it was plain wrong.

I became increasingly angry. Every week, expectant parents are given new things to worry about. Pregnant women mustn't eat too much, as it may raise the baby's risk of obesity or diabetes, but we mustn't diet, as that could have a similar effect. Neither can we exercise, for fear of triggering a miscarriage. It's enough to raise your blood pressure just thinking about it, only we mustn't get stressed, because that's bad for the baby, too. And if we do get stressed, we can't drink alcohol, go for a spa treatment, or lie on our back to relax.

It doesn't get much better once the baby is born. Before having a first child, most of us have never been left alone with a newborn, let alone been handed sole responsibility for its survival and well-being. Some of us get through it on instinct, while others consult every baby book ever published—but even these offer conflicting advice on key topics like sleep, feeding, and crying. Most books are written by people with years of experience, but did anyone systematically compare the techniques they recommended and figure out if one was better than another—or if they may be harmful to some babies? I wanted to find out.

Bumpology is my attempt to make sense of all the conflicting advice that's out there about pregnancy, birth, and raising babies. I am not a doctor, so none of what I write is intended as medical advice—although you may find it useful to refer doctors and midwives to some of the studies I cite in the Notes section. What I do have experience of is wading through the scientific research and asking questions of doctors and scientists in an attempt to make sense of it all.

The first thing to understand is that many of the newspaper headlines we read are based on one study, often preliminary, sometimes conducted on animals. Although it's in the nature of journalism to simplify, sometimes this has the unfortunate consequence that readers take what journalists write (or how their editors choose to spin it) too seriously. My husband—a fellow science journalist—has an anecdote about when he went to see a nurse to have his sperm count tested for a feature he was writing. He was told that he should avoid using his laptop on his lap, as the heat it generates could damage the quality of his sperm. When he asked the source of this advice, his own story in *The Daily Telegraph* was quoted back at him. It was based on preliminary research presented at a scientific conference on a slow news day. Although he had written some of these caveats into the original article, they had been lost in translation.

Then there are times when advice is offered for the benefit of a population rather than individuals within that population. This is particularly true of guidance issued by global bodies such as the World Health Organization, which are doing their best by women in a whole host of different economic and social situations. Telling women that they need to breast-feed for two years may save the lives of many infants in developing countries through the protection it affords against infectious disease, but it risks causing unnecessary anxiety among women in Western countries who perhaps can't breast-feed or who stop after a couple of months because they need to return to work. Advice also tends to be aimed at the *average* individual, without taking into account specific needs and circumstances.

It is important to understand that science doesn't yet have a definitive answer to many questions, even though plenty of research may have been done. Take the question of how much alcohol it's safe to drink during pregnancy. We know that there are defined risks above a certain threshold, but below this, there's a gray zone where the evidence may be mixed or conflicting. In other cases, such as eating peanuts, soaking in a Jacuzzi, or exercising, there may be a theoretical risk, but there's very little good-quality evidence to support it.

Faced with such uncertainty, many doctors and health organizations will err on the side of caution: Hence the long lists of things that pregnant women should avoid. You can't blame them; they don't want to give the wrong advice and risk someone getting sick (or worse) as a result. Yet it is my strong belief that women (and men) should be equipped with the facts they need to weigh risks and make decisions for themselves.

So how should one go about making sense of alarming newspaper headlines and statistics such as "Mom's pregnancy weight may increase risk of autism, developmental disorders"?

One thing to look for is the size of the study. If it has been conducted with fewer than a hundred people, I'd be tempted to regard the results as provisional at best; if with hundreds or thousands of people, it may be more reliable—although that also depends on what is being measured. If it's a relatively rare event such as death during childbirth, then ideally, you'd want to see a study of many thousands of people, as this should increase your confidence that the finding isn't down to chance.

Unfortunately, many of the studies I examined during the research for *Bumpology* fell into the "tens to hundreds of people" category. In some cases, this was the only evidence that existed, so it was all I had to go on, and I have tried to make that clear to the reader. In other cases, plenty of small studies had been done, but they reached conflicting conclusions; here, I have generally turned to systematic reviews in which the results of lots of studies are pooled, in order to paint as broad a picture of the evidence as possible. The highly respected Cochrane Collaboration is an international network of researchers who specialize in doing just that, and they have reviewed many of the key topics, particularly in the area of childbirth. Finally, some words about risk and statistics. Often newspapers will quote research that found an X percent increased risk of something (typically awful) happening. What they're usually referring to is the relative risk, which tends to paint a far scarier picture than the figure we really care about: the absolute risk. For example, you may be told that women who request epidural pain relief during labor are 42 percent more likely to need additional help delivering their babies (through the use of forceps or a vacuum device called a ventouse). However, the risk of needing an instrumental delivery among the general population is pretty low (around 12 percent), so what we're actually talking about is an increase of 42 percent of that 12 percent, or only a 5 percent increased risk. Another way to look at it is that for every twenty women who request epidural pain relief, there will be one extra instrumental delivery.

When you're weighing risks, it's sensible to ask yourself a couple of questions. First what is the risk of the bad thing happening to start with, and just how serious are the consequences if it does happen? Second, how much does the action you're considering increase that risk? Finally, how great is the benefit if you decide to do it anyway?

In writing this book, I have tried to cut through some of the confusion and conflicting advice, leaving parents with the facts about the state of the scientific evidence. It is for individual parents to decide how much risk they want to take and what is going to work best in their circumstances. Having a baby can be one of the greatest joys that life bestows, but it is hard work. We can do without any unnecessary guilt, anxiety, and doubt.

It's also a time of great wonder. I still find it staggering that a single egg and sperm can meet and trigger the cascade of events that lead to a new little person being built and then unfolding into this fascinating, lovable, and endlessly entertaining individual. In researching this book, I've learned things about babies that will never cease to amaze me—indeed, I may never look at my children in the same way again.

ONE

BUMP

Food and Drink

. 1 .
Why do pregnant women crave unhealthy food?

Angelina Jolie craved chocolate with cinnamon and chile, Cate Blanchett wanted pickles and ice cream, while Britney Spears is said to have wanted to eat soil. A recent study on the pregnancy website www.babycenter.com found that about 85 percent of American women experienced at least one food craving during pregnancy. Around 40 percent craved sweet foods, while 33 percent lusted after salty snacks. Spicy foods came in third, at 17 percent, followed by fresh fruit, at 10 percent.

Surprisingly few scientific studies have been carried out on food cravings during pregnancy. Those that have been find that pregnant women often have a desire for salty foods and become less sensitive to the taste, as well as becoming more sensitive to bitter tastes.

The salt craving may come about because, as their blood volume expands, pregnant women need slightly more salt to maintain the balance of fluids in their bodies. An aversion to bitter flavors is less easy to explain, but some have proposed that it steers women away from poisonous plants, which are often bitter (see 3: "What causes morning sickness?").

As to why pregnant women crave sweet foods, studies of how taste preferences vary over the menstrual cycle may provide some clues. Women tend to want foods that are high in carbohydrates and fat during the second half of the menstrual cycle, when levels of the hormone progesterone are high. They are more sensitive to sweet tastes during the first half of the cycle, when levels of estrogen are higher.

Although both hormones increase during pregnancy, there is relatively more progesterone than estrogen, which may explain why women long for sweet, energy-rich foods like chocolate or cake (or preferably both at the same time).

A lot of people assume that you crave the foods your body needs. Although no one has studied this specifically in pregnant women, there is some evidence that it may be true. Leigh Gibson and his colleagues at the University of Roehampton, London, gave their test group two flavors of soup to try: one that was high in protein and one that was low. A few days later, the volunteers were either starved of protein or given a protein-rich drink before being offered a choice of the two soups for lunch. Those who were protein-starved said they preferred the protein-rich flavor, and they also ate far more of it. In other words, if you are starved of protein, you subconsciously begin to prefer the taste of foods that contain large amounts of it. "It seems we can rapidly learn to want to eat foods that supply needed nutrients like protein," says Gibson.

Likewise, cravings for sweet, fatty foods may reflect a need for energy, although Gibson cautions that they could also reflect a need for emotional comfort, as we often get a lot of pleasure from eating them. So if your body is screaming out for ice cream, perhaps it's worth considering how much you've already eaten that day before concluding that your baby is deficient in chocolate-chip cookie dough.

. 2 .

Do pregnant women really eat coal?

"Have you been eating coal?" was the first thing my dad asked me upon learning I was pregnant. Strange as it sounds, some women develop a taste for minerals, metallic objects, and even soil during pregnancy, a phenomenon known as pica. Some have proposed that it's a sign of iron deficiency—though how much iron you'd get from a mouthful of coal is questionable.

A survey of 2,231 British women found that 31 percent claimed to have experienced unusual cravings during pregnancy. At the top of the list was ice, followed by coal, toothpaste, sponges, mud, chalk, laundry soap, matches, and rubber. One of my neighbors even reported a penchant for cigarette ash during her pregnancy.

Many of these phenomena have their own names. Pagophagia, or ice-eating, is common among American women as well: A separate survey found that 18 percent of women in the state of Georgia did it, the amount they ate ranging from a couple of glasses of ice cubes to several pounds a day.

Earth-eating, or geophagia, is particularly common in African countries such as Tanzania, where up to 60 percent of pregnant women indulge. Clay-rich soil seems particularly desirable, although pottery is sometimes eaten instead.

Scientists have proposed various explanations for pica, including cultural trends, stress relief (like biting one's fingernails), and hunger. Some women who have been interviewed about their pica say that it helps to relieve heartburn and nausea, and often the items they choose have an alkaline pH, which may help to neutralize stomach acid. Most women, though, have no idea why they crave such oddities.

A common scientific explanation is that these women are deficient in certain nutrients, such as iron, zinc, or calcium. Although there have been hundreds of reports of iron-deficient women craving soil and other pica, when researchers have analyzed how much iron is released from the digestion of soil or clay, the answer is: very little. Neither does giving women iron supplements to cure their anemia stop their cravings. What's more, eating clay and soil can actually inhibit the uptake of iron and other minerals by the gut. But just because soil doesn't cure anemia doesn't mean that anemia doesn't trigger the craving. "It may be that being deficient in essential minerals induces a craving for anything mineral-tasting," says Gibson.

An intriguing suggestion is that eating clay reduces the chances of food poisoning. Several studies have shown that certain substances in soil can bind to bacteria, viruses, and toxins in the gut, preventing them from being absorbed into the bloodstream. Some types of clay also seem to increase the secretion of mucus in the intestines, making it harder for bacteria to get through.

Why women crave ice remains a mystery. Some have suggested that it has the same crunchy texture as dry clay or soil, so eating it has a similar psychological effect. Others propose that it calms tongue pain or swelling, which is a common symptom of iron deficiency.

. 3 .
What causes morning sickness?

I write this in the throes of morning sickness, seven weeks pregnant and curled up in bed with a hot-water bottle, praying for the current wave of nausea to pass. This is my second pregnancy, and I'm sure it's worse this time (for one thing, I'm actually vomiting, rather than just feeling queasy).

Up to 80 percent of women experience some degree of morning sickness during pregnancy. Generally, it is at its worst between weeks four and ten, and even the unlucky few who continue to feel sick after ten weeks are usually free of it by week twenty.

There are several theories about why morning sickness should exist. One is that it evolved to steer pregnant women away from eating plants containing toxins that might harm the baby (it's also why pregnant women are thought to develop an aversion to bitter foods; see 1: "Why do pregnant women crave unhealthy food?"). But in that case, you'd expect women to feel sicker after they'd eaten fruit or vegetables, and there's little evidence to support this, although I did develop a weird aversion to lettuce in my first pregnancy. The theory is also dealt a minor blow by the fact that India (where many people are vegetarian) has the lowest rate of morning sickness, with just 35 percent of women suffering from it. Japan has the highest rate, with 84 percent of pregnant women experiencing nausea and vomiting.

A related theory is that morning sickness evolved to protect the embryo from bacteria or parasites in the diet that could harm it. Paul Sherman and Samuel Flaxman at Cornell University put forward this theory after reviewing studies involving nearly eighty thousand pregnant women from around the world. Pregnant women are particularly susceptible to food poisoning because their immune systems are suppressed, and serious illness can increase the risk of stillbirth or miscarriage (one reason why we're told to avoid soft cheeses). Cells in the embryo are also dividing rapidly, leaving them more susceptible to any damage to DNA caused by harmful toxins.

Sherman and Flaxman note that the level of nausea and vomiting usually peaks at the same time the baby's vital organs are forming, and a baby is also growing very quickly at this point, so if its DNA is damaged, that could have disastrous effects. Commonly avoided foods include meat, fish, poultry, and eggs (foods that are the most likely to contain dangerous microorganisms), as well as caffeinated drinks like tea or coffee, which could harm the baby if consumed in large amounts.

It's true that morning sickness is less common in societies that consume only small amounts of meat and fish and eat more plants as staple foods, including some American Indian and First Nations tribes. Women experiencing morning sickness may also be marginally less likely to miscarry. One large study found that 90 percent of women with no morning sickness gave birth to a live baby, compared to 96 percent of women who did experience morning sickness.

Perhaps more convincingly, morning sickness may simply be an unfortunate side effect of the same hormone that confirmed you were pregnant in the first place. Human chorionic gonadotropin (HCG), the hormone detected by pregnancy tests, is produced by the embryo during the early weeks of pregnancy in order to maintain a structure called the corpus luteum, which produces other pregnancy hormones needed to keep the lining of the uterus nice and thick until the placenta is big enough to take over. But HCG has other effects on the body, such as stimulating the thyroid gland in the neck. This gland produces several hormones that regulate metabolism, and high levels of thyroid hormones seem to be associated with particularly severe vomiting in women with morning sickness. Two other pregnancy hormones, progesterone and estrogen, may also contribute to general feelings of queasiness, bloating, and heartburn, as they slow down the digestive system, so food takes longer to travel through your gut. Rampaging progesterone may explain another annoying side effect of early pregnancy: extreme tiredness. At very high doses, progesterone can be used as an anesthetic, having a similar effect on the brain to barbiturates.

No one has shown conclusively that women with higher levels of these hormones are more prone to morning sickness; it's just a theory. Neither do we know why some babies seem to cause more sickness than others— although the placentas of female fetuses do seem to produce more HCG than those of male fetuses (presumably because hormone production is linked to the X chromosome). Just three weeks into pregnancy, HCG levels are nearly a fifth higher in women carrying female embryos than those carrying males. There is also some evidence that women with particularly severe morning sickness are marginally more likely to be carrying girls or twins.

. 4 .
Is there anything I can do to reduce morning sickness?

Perhaps, although the evidence isn't very strong. Both the American College of Obstetrics and Gynecology (ACOG) and the UK's National Institute for Health and Clinical Excellence (NICE), which offers evidence-based guidance to doctors, suggest that ginger may help to relieve nausea and vomiting. ACOG also recommends vitamin B6, or vitamin B6 plus an antihistamine called doxylamine.

However, the Cochrane Collaboration recently reviewed the evidence for morning-sickness treatments, including acupuncture, acupressure, vitamin B6, ginger, and some anti-sickness drugs, and found little consistent or reliable evidence to support any of them. You may just have to ride out the sickness and look forward to the later stages of pregnancy, when you'll be carrying a proud bump and should be able to feel your baby moving about inside you.

. 5 .
How much alcohol is it safe to drink during pregnancy?

I'm sure I'm not alone in feeling confused and a little irritated by the messages women are given about alcohol consumption during pregnancy. A recent discussion on the UK Internet forum Mumsnet about whether someone could indulge in a few glasses of wine at a wedding generated sixty-nine responses—with angry arguments on both sides.

A withering list of countries—including the U.S., UK, France, Canada, Australia, New Zealand, Ireland, the Netherlands, and Spain—currently advise pregnant women to abstain completely from alcohol during pregnancy (although the UK government concedes that if you do decide to drink, you should "consume no more than one to two units, or 10–20 milliliters, once or twice a week"). The U.S. advises women who are even thinking about getting pregnant to abstain.

Yet until quite recently, pregnant women were told to drink half a pint of Guinness or stout each night to keep their iron levels up. We all know of women who have drunk moderate amounts of alcohol during pregnancy—or who have been blind drunk before realizing they were pregnant—and their babies appear to have turned out fine.

So what is a safe amount of alcohol to drink? When researchers at the UK's National Perinatal Epidemiology Unit in Oxford reviewed forty-six scientific papers looking at the effects of low to moderate drinking during pregnancy, they found no increased risk of miscarriage, stillbirth, premature birth, low birth weight, or birth defects (including fetal alcohol syndrome). These women were drinking a fair amount of alcohol each week—up to 10.4 units per week, or about five small glasses of wine. However, the researchers also found plenty of flaws in the studies, which meant they couldn't say conclusively that light to moderate drinking is safe.

The truth is that no one really knows what constitutes a "safe" amount of alcohol. It's clear that large amounts can cause fetal alcohol syndrome (FAS), a serious condition that stunts the physical and mental development of the child. According to a report by the UK's Royal College of Obstetricians and Gynaecologists, drinking more than six units a day puts babies at risk of FAS and can also trigger miscarriage. Birth defects are three times more common in the babies of women who drink more than four and a half units a day, compared to light drinkers and abstainers—but birth defects are still pretty rare. Meanwhile, 45 percent of women who drink more than two units (a small glass of wine) a day during their third trimester may have a baby with low birth weight, which can increase the risk of developmental or behavioral problems later in life—although the evidence for this is mixed.

However, below this level there's a big gray zone in which there may or may not be an effect. In 2012, a large Danish study concluded that one to eight drinks a week seemed to have had no effect on children's IQ or attention span, or on brain functions such as planning, organization, and self-control by the time they reached the age of five. Unlike many studies, this one was well designed, in that it asked women how much alcohol they were drinking when they were actually pregnant, then followed the progress of their children as they grew older.

It's also not correct to assume that abstinence is the best policy: Several studies have suggested that children born to mothers who drank one to two units of alcohol per week in their pregnancy were less likely to have behavioral problems than those born to abstainers. In one such study, the sons of light drinkers had fewer behavioral troubles and less hyperactivity, and the daughters had fewer peer problems and emotional difficulties. Children of moderate drinkers, who consumed three to six units per week, were broadly similar to those of women who drank nothing, while there were slightly more behavioral problems in the children of women who drank more than seven units a week. However, it's also possible that these differences arose because light drinkers were more relaxed, or came from higher-income or more educated backgrounds than abstainers.

Patrick O'Brien of the RCOG says that light drinking—one to two units once or twice a week—is extremely unlikely to harm your baby. Vivian Nathanson of the British Medical Association (which advocates abstinence) admits that up to eight units is unlikely to cause harm, but suggests it is far better to err on the side of caution and drink nothing or very little.

However, there may be other reasons why women are told to abstain. One is that it's very difficult to do broad enough studies on light drinkers to catch the very small number of problems that might crop up. It's possible that light drinking does carry a small risk, but we just don't know about it yet. Another is that women are not trusted to be capable of following guidelines on a recommended number of units. "We know that a lot of people drink a great deal more than they think they do, because what they think is a unit is in fact several units," says Nathanson. "Abstinence is an easy thing to measure."

It's also likely that babies are more vulnerable to the effects of alcohol at some periods of their development than at others. One recent study found that drinking more than one alcoholic drink per day during pregnancy generally increased the risk of babies being underweight or shorter in length at birth, but consuming alcohol between weeks seven and twelve was strongly linked with the characteristic deformities associated with fetal alcohol syndrome: small head, small upper jaw, thin upper lip, and small, narrow eyes.

Women who had just a couple of sips of alcohol were classified as nondrinkers, however. Weeks seven to twelve of pregnancy are particularly busy in terms of development: In just five weeks, the baby goes from looking like a mutant tadpole to looking like a human being, while after week twelve, its main task is to get bigger. So perhaps it's no surprise that this would be a particularly critical time to avoid anything that might perturb that development. It's also probably the time when women are least likely to want to drink, as morning sickness is at its peak and most women will be feeling dog-tired.

Ultimately, every woman needs to decide for herself whether she believes the occasional drink during pregnancy is okay. Based on the evidence I've seen, I've developed my own set of rules.

- The first trimester is when the baby is most at risk, so try to avoid drinking then. If you didn't realize you were pregnant, just stop drinking now. Most women realize they are pregnant by seven weeks, which is when the most critical point seems to start.
- If abstinence isn't for you, try to stick to one to two units once or twice a week. However, if you occasionally drink more than this (up to about eight units a week), it's probably fine.
- Know how much a unit of alcohol is, and remember that some wines and beers are stronger than others.

- Binge drinking is likely to be worse than drinking the same amount over a long period because it exposes your baby to higher concentrations of alcohol. So try to spread your drinks out as much as possible.

. 6 .
Can unborn babies taste what Mom is eating?

Unborn babies are floating in a veritable cocktail of taste sensations, which may be teaching them what's good to eat in preparation for when they pop out into the big wide world.

Taste buds on the tongue begin to develop just thirteen to fifteen weeks into pregnancy, enabling babies to detect simple tastes such as sweet, sour, and salty, but many of the more complex flavors we experience are the result of volatile molecules from foods like garlic passing over smell receptors in the nose.

All of these things can find their way into the amniotic fluid that surrounds the baby, in much the same way that flavors get into breast milk (see 111: "Does what I eat change the flavor of my milk?"). "If it gets into the blood supply, it will get into the amniotic fluid and the breast milk," says Julie Mennella at the Monell Chemical Senses Center in Philadelphia, who spends her days trying to understand how preferences for certain flavors develop.

During the third trimester of pregnancy, fetuses breathe and swallow around a liter of amniotic fluid a day—probably as practice for when they're born, rather than for any nutrients—and much of this fluid will pass smell and taste receptors in the nose and mouth. Some smelly molecules, such as the sulfurous compounds that give garlic its characteristic smell and taste, are so potent that if you take a sample of amniotic fluid from a woman who has eaten a garlicky meal, you can smell the garlic wafting from it.

So unborn babies do get a taste of what their moms are eating during pregnancy, and they also seem to remember it. Several studies have shown that babies whose mothers ate a lot of garlic or aniseed during pregnancy are

attracted to those smells in the first days after birth, making rooting or sucking motions when they catch their scent.

. 7 .
Can Mom's food fads influence her baby's palate?

Not only are babies treated to a banquet of flavors before birth, it seems
the memory of these tastes may influence the kinds of foods they like in later
life.

Studies have shown that if Mom drinks a glass of carrot juice four times a
week during the last trimester of pregnancy or the first two months of breast-
feeding, her baby will find cereal prepared with carrot juice particularly ap-
pealing once it has been weaned. Babies whose moms eat a lot of fruit during
pregnancy are also more likely to enjoy fruit during weaning. "The baby is
learning what foods Mom likes," says Mennella. "I think it's the first way they
learn what foods are safe and also what foods are available."

Trying to eat as many different flavors as possible during pregnancy and
breast-feeding should therefore expose your baby to a smorgasbord of different tastes, and in theory, this may make them less prone to fussy eating.
However, it could also set a bad example if you choose to indulge in less
wholesome options. Babies whose mothers drank two small glasses of wine
a week during pregnancy showed more smiling, suckling, and licking expressions in response to the smell of alcohol than those whose moms drank very
little or nothing at all. It's not clear whether this penchant for alcohol lasted
into adulthood, though a bizarre study on rats suggests it might. Adolescent
rats whose mothers had consumed alcohol during pregnancy showed a greater
interest in drunken partners than those whose mothers hadn't consumed alcohol—presumably because they could smell the alcohol on their breath.

It gets even weirder. Several studies have found that children's propensity
for salt can be influenced by the degree of morning sickness their mothers
experienced. Sixteen-week-old babies whose mothers endured moderate to
severe vomiting during the first fourteen weeks of pregnancy were more toler-

ant of salty drinks than those whose mothers experienced no morning sickness. One possible explanation is that throwing up can dehydrate women, making their amniotic fluid more concentrated and salty.

. 8 .
Is coffee bad for my baby?

If you're someone who simply can't function without the morning latte or espresso, the great news is you don't have to stop. Although a handful of studies have linked the consumption of caffeine to reduced birth weight and an increased risk of preterm birth or stillbirth, other studies have found no effect.

The Cochrane Collaboration tries to make sense of these kinds of contradictory studies by taking a bunch of them and systematically weighing the evidence to help people make informed decisions about their health. It recently weighed in on the issue of caffeine during pregnancy and concluded that drinking three cups of instant caffeinated coffee a day during early pregnancy probably has no effect, so there is no reason to avoid it in small amounts.

Drinking a lot more than three cups of coffee a day may be more of a problem, however. One large study found that women who drank more than 550 milligrams of caffeine a day (roughly equivalent to six regular cups of coffee, or twelve cups of tea or green tea) had slightly shorter babies.

If you do decide to drink coffee, one thing to watch for is that different blends vary in the amount of caffeine they contain. In the U.S. and the UK, pregnant women are advised to limit themselves to 200 milligrams of caffeine a day—somewhere between two and four cups of coffee, depending on whose data you use. But a recent survey of espressos bought in Scotland found a sixfold variation in the amount of caffeine they contained, with one espresso bought in Glasgow's West End containing 322 milligrams. A Starbucks espresso, by contrast, contained just 51 milligrams. Since lattes and cappuccinos are often made by diluting a double shot of espresso, you might want to ask your barista to hold the second shot.

As a rough guide, here's what the FDA says about how much caffeine common food and drinks contain:

- One cup (5 oz.) of coffee: 60–150 mg. caffeine
- One cup (5 oz.) of decaf coffee: 2–5 mg caffeine
- One cup (5 oz.) of tea: 40–80 mg caffeine
- One can (12 oz.) of Coca-Cola: 64 mg caffeine
- One can (12 oz.) of Diet Coke: 45 mg caffeine
- One 1 oz. bar of plain (bittersweet) chocolate: 5–35 mg caffeine
- One 1 oz. bar of milk chocolate: 1–15 mg caffeine

. 9 .
Can I eat peanuts during pregnancy?

The official advice on this waxes and wanes, but currently, both the American Academy of Pediatrics (AAP) and the UK Food Standards Agency say that it's fine to eat peanuts during pregnancy (even though both previously advised against it if there was a history of allergy or asthma in the child's immediate family).

Certainly, several studies have suggested an indirect link between eating peanuts during pregnancy and childhood allergy. For example, in 2010, many newspapers seized upon an American study that found that children were more likely to test positive for antibodies against peanuts if their mothers had eaten peanut products during pregnancy (an indirect marker for possible peanut allergy). However, even the study's authors urged caution in interpreting its results. For one thing, they relied on mothers' memories of how many peanuts they had eaten, rather than measuring quantities themselves. They also tested only children who already had suspected allergies to milk or eggs rather than the general population, and they didn't test for peanut allergy directly.

What's more, several studies have found the opposite: that eating peanuts during pregnancy may protect infants against allergies. In such situations, the most sensible thing to do is to weigh the results of as many studies as possible to decide where the best evidence lies. Fortunately, someone has done this for us: In 2008, the American Academy of Pediatrics reviewed the available studies and concluded that there currently isn't enough evidence to support the idea that avoiding peanuts—or other foods—during pregnancy will reduce your child's risk of allergies. A recent review by the UK's Committee on Toxicology reached a similar conclusion. This doesn't necessarily mean peanuts have the all-clear; just that more good-quality research is needed to decide either way. Until then, you may as well carry on eating peanut butter—spread it on pickles, if you'd like.

. 10 .
Should pregnant women really eat for two?

There's no doubt that being pregnant is hungry work, and no, you're not just being greedy: The hormone progesterone, which soars during pregnancy, is known to boost the appetite. But although it can be tempting to help yourself to a second slice of cake because you're "eating for two," there are good reasons not to overindulge—at least not every day. The good news is that if you can't resist, it is generally safe to exercise during pregnancy (see 22: "Is it safe to exercise during pregnancy?").

In 2009, the U.S. Institute of Medicine issued guidelines saying that women should gain no more than 25 to 35 pounds during pregnancy, while those who are already overweight should gain no more than 15 to 25 pounds, and obese women no more than 11 to 20 pounds.

That's all very well, but around half of women gain more weight than this, and although a little extra weight is unlikely to harm you or your baby, putting on a lot of extra weight can increase your risk of gestational diabetes, high blood pressure, and needing a C-section or mechanical help (like forceps) to get the baby out.

Another good reason not to overindulge is that women who put on a lot of extra weight during pregnancy find it harder to shift it afterward—and I speak from bitter experience. A recent review of nine studies found that women who gained more than the recommended amount of weight carried an average extra 3.06 kilograms (6.75 pounds) three years after giving birth and an extra 4.72 kilograms (10.4 pounds) after fifteen years. Putting on too much weight too quickly may also increase your chances of having hemorrhoids, varicose veins, and stretch marks.

So how many extra calories does your body need to grow a baby? Most doctors recommend eating just 100 to 300 extra calories a day during pregnancy, which doesn't add up to even a slice of cake.

As a rough guide, you should expect to put on 2 to 4 pounds in total during the first twelve weeks, then 1 to 2 pounds a week after that.

. 11 .
How dangerous is it to eat Camembert and blue cheese?

Why is it that, when you're pregnant, beautiful creamy soft cheese is everywhere? And yet we can't eat it—we're told—because soft and blue-veined varieties of cheese carry a risk of listeriosis, a type of food poisoning that can trigger birth defects and miscarriage. Listeriosis is caused by a bacterium called *Listeria monocytogenes,* which is present in soil and therefore gets on the grass eaten by the cows, sheep, and goats that produce the milk for cheese-making. These bacteria are usually destroyed by heating or pasteurization, but if they do survive, they find it easier to grow in ripened soft and blue-veined cheeses, which are often less acidic and contain more moisture than hard cheeses.

Although people can come into contact with listeria without getting listeriosis, pregnant women are twenty times more likely to develop it than nonpregnant women of the same age because their immune systems are weakened. Even so, cases of listeriosis are pretty rare. According to the Centers for Disease Control and Prevention (CDC), there are around 1,600 cases in the U.S. a year (resulting in around 500 deaths), and only around 17 percent of these cases are in pregnant women. People over the age of sixty are also at increased risk, as are people with cancer or any other disease that suppresses the immune system.

That said, the consequences of listeria infection during pregnancy are pretty terrifying. Around one in 25,000 pregnant women contracts listeriosis, and besides making the woman feel rotten, the infection can cause complications and trigger miscarriage in around 20 percent of cases.

Unfortunately, we can't say how many cases of listeriosis there would be if pregnant women decided to ignore the standard advice and scoff artisan cheeses at will. But cheese isn't the only source of listeria infection—prepacked sandwiches, ready-to-eat meats such as hot dogs, sliced meat and pâté, butter, and smoked salmon can also carry the bug, so if you're worried about listeria, you should probably avoid these as well. A recent analysis of the likely sources of listeria infection in the U.S. found that melons and hummus were prime suspects, as was living on a cattle farm, while a review of recent UK cases found that foods such as prepacked sandwiches or ready-to-eat salads topped the list of likely sources of infection.

The good news is that thoroughly cooking risky foods should kill the bacteria that cause listeriosis—as long as you ensure that the food is piping hot before serving. There are mixed messages about whether soft cheese made from pasteurized milk is safe. The CDC says it is, while the UK's NHS cautions against eating soft cheese, regardless of whether it says it has been pasteurized. Pasteurization will kill any bugs that were living in the milk before it was treated, so that should reduce the risk, but there is still a chance that cheese could become contaminated during packaging.

The Pregnant Body

. 12 .
Can the shape of my bump or anything else predict the gender of my child?

A belly like a basketball, bad morning sickness, weird food cravings . . . If you believe the old wives' tales, you're definitely expecting a boy. But are any of these guessing games underpinned by scientific evidence?

Let's take a look.

Women who have basketball-shaped bumps are expecting boys

Women who carry high and all up front are expecting boys, while a low, wide bump is a sign of a girl—or so says the folklore. But Janet DiPietro of Johns Hopkins University has investigated and found no correlation between the shape of a woman's bump and the sex of the child developing inside it.

She asked 104 pregnant women what gender of child they thought they were carrying, and whether they thought their bump was all up front or spread around the hips; the interviewer also made an assessment. There was only moderate agreement between the two, suggesting that the shape of a woman's bump is pretty subjective, and neither assessment correctly predicted the gender of the child who eventually popped out.

Bad morning sickness means you're having a boy

Actually, the opposite is true: Moms-to-be with really bad morning sickness are more likely to have a girl. In 1999, researchers analyzed the records of 8,186 Swedish women whose morning sickness was so bad that they had to be admitted into a hospital and found that 44.3 percent of them gave birth to boys (compared to 51.4 percent of the general population).

The researchers blame higher levels of the pregnancy hormone HCG in women carrying girls. This is the hormone that pregnancy tests detect, and it is produced at the beginning of pregnancy in order to maintain the corpus luteum, which churns out other pregnancy hormones until the placenta is developed enough to take over. No one really understands why female fetuses are associated with higher levels of HCG, but differences have been detected as early as sixteen days after fertilization and continue throughout pregnancy. HCG may be responsible for keeping pregnancies going, but it comes with some side effects. It can make your bladder overreactive and cause you to feel sick.

Shortly after this study was published in the *Lancet*, Henrik Toft Sørensen of Aarhus and Aalborg University Hospitals in Denmark wrote to the journal, claiming that marital status also influenced the sex of the baby, with fewer boys born to single mothers. Like the Swedish group, he found that women with severe morning sickness were more likely to give birth to girls, but the correlation was even stronger in single mothers. Among women with severe morning sickness, 40 percent who lived alone had boys, compared with 45 percent who lived with their partner (and 51 percent of women who didn't experience morning sickness).

Fetal heart rate predicts the baby's sex

One of the most exciting moments of pregnancy is when your doctor holds a Doppler probe to your belly and you hear your baby's heartbeat for the first time. Because fetal hearts beat much faster than adult hearts, this often sounds like galloping horses.

According to this old wives' tale, if your baby's heart rate is faster than 140 beats per minute (bpm) you're expecting a girl; if it's slower, you're expecting a boy. The trouble is that the heart rate tends to decrease during pregnancy, from 170 to 200 bpm at eight to ten weeks down to 120 to 160 bpm by mid-pregnancy, and there seems to be little difference between boys and girls—at least during early pregnancy.

In one study, researchers used ultrasound to measure heart rate in 477 fetuses before the fourteenth week of pregnancy. The average heart rate of girls was 151.7 bpm, and for boys 154.9 bpm, though this wasn't a big enough difference to be statistically significant and would be unreliable to use to guess the baby's gender.

Interestingly, a bigger difference can be detected during labor itself, when female babies do seem to have faster heart rates. The reason is unknown.

Strange food cravings mean you're having a boy

There's not much evidence to support this one, although one study did find that women who are carrying boys have bigger appetites. It recorded the eating habits of 244 pregnant women and found that those who gave birth to boys ate 10 percent more calories per day than those who had girls. The trouble is, how do you know if you're hungrier than the next pregnant mom? Indeed, the authors of this study admitted that the difference was not big enough to predict the sex of a baby with any accuracy.

Women "just know"

"Female intuition" claims power over many things—including being able to predict the sex of unborn children. And it may be one of the best tools going for predicting your baby's gender. Victor Shamas at the University of Tucson asked 108 pregnant women to guess the sex of their baby. Seventy-five of them claimed to have a gut feeling about it or had experienced a dream, and 60 percent of them were correct—which is more than you'd expect by chance. When the researchers discounted women who had a strong preference for a boy or a girl, the forty-eight remaining women guessed right 71 percent of the time. Unfortunately, the study was never published, but it does provide ammunition for women whose partners keep on suggesting ridiculous boys' names: "Sorry, darling, but I just know it's going to be a girl . . ."

If the egg implants on the right side of the uterus, it's a boy; if on the left, it's a girl

This is not so much an old wives' tale as an interesting piece of research posted on an Internet forum for obstetricians in 2007 that has generated a lot of discussion. A Canadian sonographer called Saad Ramzi Ismail reported that, based on scans of 5,376 pregnant women, he found that the position in which the placenta attaches to the uterus strongly predicts whether a woman is having a boy or a girl. He said that 97.2 percent of male fetuses attach on the right side of the uterus, while 97.5 percent of female fetuses attach on the left. Although Ramzi's work was written up as a scientific paper, it doesn't appear to have been published in any peer-reviewed journal, so his methods haven't been subjected to any detailed scientific scrutiny. Neither did he give any satisfactory explanation as to why the location of the placenta should influence the baby's gender. One earlier study by an American group suggested that women with low-lying placentas (a condition called placenta previa) were 14 percent more likely to have boys, although the biological mechanism behind this is also unclear. One possibility is that the time of conception might influence where in the uterus an embryo implants (as there's some evidence that boys are more likely to be conceived if you have sex at the time of ovulation; see 149: "Is there anything I can do to influence the gender of my baby?"). Alternatively, temperature differences in different areas of the uterus might better favor the survival of male or female embryos. In 2010, an Australian group announced at the World Congress on Ultrasound in Obstetrics and Gynecology that they had tried to replicate Ramzi's findings. They recorded placental location in 277 women and found no convincing evidence that it correlated with the sex of the baby.

. 13 .
Why don't pregnant women topple over?

Every year, a magazine called the *Annals of Improbable Research* awards the Ig Nobels Prizes, which celebrate the unusual, honor the imaginative, and spur people's interest in science, medicine, and technology. In October 2009, the physics prize went to a group of anthropologists who dared to ask the question: "Why don't pregnant women topple over?"

As a woman's body grows during pregnancy and her bump begins to stick out, this changes her center of gravity, making her more clumsy and prone to waddling. But it's rare to see a pregnant woman topple over—even on London's Tube system, where few people are willing to stand up and offer her a seat.

The reason, found Katherine Whitcome and her colleagues at the University of Cincinnati, is down to the shape of the spine. The bones in women's lower backs are more wedge-shaped than men's, making it easier for the backbone to bend. The bony projections surrounding each little bone are also relatively larger in women, providing additional support to the spine. Because of this, women's spines have a more pronounced curvature than men's, which allows them to shift the upper half of the body backward during pregnancy and counterbalance the weight of the growing baby.

. 14 .
Why do women get a linea nigra and other brown patches on their skin during pregnancy?

The linea nigra is a brownish line extending from the belly button down to below the panty line that appears in most women during pregnancy and remains for about a year after the birth. It corresponds to a line of collagen-rich connective tissue called the linea alba, which separates the abdominal muscles and is what underlies the "six-pack" you sometimes see in fit, muscular people.

One annoying side effect of rampaging pregnancy hormones such as estrogen and progesterone is that they cause skin cells called melanocytes to churn out more of the brown pigment melanin (the same thing that makes you turn brown in the sun). These melanocytes are naturally more common in some areas of the body than others, including around previous areas of sun damage and along the lower half of the linea alba, which can leave many women with uneven patches of brown skin (also known as the mask of pregnancy) and this characteristic brown line running down their bellies.

Just why these cells should choose to hang out along the linea alba is unknown, but one theory is that many of them simply become stuck here during embryonic development, when they migrate out of a structure called the neural crest, which runs down the middle of the embryo's body.

The mask of pregnancy usually disappears after pregnancy, but you can prevent it from developing in the first place by wearing a good sunscreen containing both UVA and UVB protection.

Another irritation of pregnancy is that estrogen combined with an increase in blood volume causes the growth of new blood vessels, and this can give rise to spider veins—small red branches on the surface of the skin. Most spider veins should fade after giving birth, but some may stubbornly remain. If they make you really unhappy, they can be removed with simple laser treatment, but it's probably worth waiting until your childbearing days are over, as you're likely to get more in subsequent pregnancies.

Added pressure from the unborn baby on the veins that return blood from the legs to the heart can also cause varicose veins, which afflict around 40 percent of pregnant women. Elasticated stockings, sleeping on the left side of your body, light exercise, elevating your legs in the air, and avoiding standing or sitting for long amounts of time can all reduce the chances of them developing.

. 15 .
Is there anything I can do to prevent stretch marks?

My waist grew fourteen inches during the course of my first pregnancy— not quite a doubling of its pre-pregnancy size, but if we assume the height of a pregnant bump is around six inches, that's a sizable increase. What's incredible is that you don't grow any new skin to do this; it's achieved simply through the stretching of existing skin. Hormones including estrogen and relaxin cause the collagen fibers that give skin its elasticity to become less sticky, so they can be pulled apart as the baby grows. Unfortunately, if this process happens too quickly, the result is stretch marks—a form of scarring. One recent study found that women with low levels of relaxin were more prone to stretch marks, possibly because their connective tissue was less elastic and therefore more prone to scarring. If you get through pregnancy without any stretch marks, you're in the lucky minority—particularly if you have white skin, which shows stretch marks more clearly.

Your susceptibility to stretch marks is dictated by your genetics and how quickly you grow, so you should try to keep weight gain as slow and steady as possible. Having strong abdominal muscles should also reduce the rate at which your bump pops out and therefore how quickly the skin stretches, adds Jenny Murase, a dermatologist at the University of California in San Francisco.

Many women try rubbing oil or cocoa butter into their bumps to ward off stretch marks, and several recent studies have set out to investigate whether this works. One, which analyzed results in women who rubbed olive oil into their bumps twice a day for eight weeks during their second and third trimesters, found no significant difference in stretch marks compared to women who did nothing. Two other studies, which compared women who rubbed cocoa butter on their bumps with those who applied a standard moisturizer, found no difference.

Even if moisturizing doesn't prevent stretch marks, it may speed up their disappearance, says Murase. "For my own pregnancy, I used cocoa butter on my abdomen, even though there's no good published evidence that I'm aware of," she says. "Stretch marks are often reddened at first, and if the skin is overly dry, it may be more irritated and take longer for that redness to fade, so I think it's a good practice to use moisturizer."

There may yet be some hope in a cream called Trofolastin, which reduced the occurrence of stretch marks in women who applied it daily from week twelve of pregnancy, compared to those who used a placebo cream. According to the study, 56 percent of women using the placebo developed stretch marks, against 34 percent of those who used Trofolastin (which is marketed by the European company Novartis and is available online). It contains vitamin E, collagen, elastin, and extracts of a plant used in traditional Asian medicine called Gotu kola (*Centella asiatica*).

Another preliminary study suggests that women with higher levels of vitamin C in their bodies during late pregnancy are less likely to have stretch marks. However, since several studies have linked vitamin C supplements to preterm birth, it may be wiser to eat a healthy and balanced diet with plenty of fruit and vegetables than to cram yourself with vitamin C tablets.

. 16 .
Do big parents have bigger babies?

What do you get if you cross a male Shire horse with a female Shetland pony? If you're wincing at the very thought, the answer is a Shetland-sized foal that the mother can push out without being torn in two. Women with strapping partners needn't worry about how their brute of a child will fit through their narrow hips, because women have the greater say over the size of the baby they'll produce—at least up until the point of birth.

It was back in 1938 that researchers first thought of crossing Shire horses with Shetland ponies in order to see what happened. They found that when a female Shire horse was mated with a male Shetland pony, the foal was bigger than a purely Shetland foal but smaller than a purely Shire foal. But when a female Shetland pony was mated with a male Shire horse, the foal weighed the same as a purebred Shetland foal. In other words, something was happening in the uterus of the female horse to control the foal's growth so it ended up in proportion to the mother's size. Of course, this is sensible from an evolutionary point of view; otherwise, many more women with large partners would have perished in labor, along with their babies.

More recently, the use of donor eggs and surrogacy to help infertile couples has shown that the newborn's size bears more relation to that of the biological mother, rather than that of the father or surrogate mother.

The current best guess of what's happening is that even though the fetus inherits a set of genes from both the mother and the father, the way they are expressed is not random, and in some situations, the mother's genes take precedence and veto the father's genes. Generally, the mother's genes are thought to influence the size of the fetus, while the father's control the development of the placenta.

But Mom's diet can also influence how big her baby grows. On average, babies weigh an extra .4 oz for every pound a mother gains on top of the recommended weight gain of 25 to 35 pounds during pregnancy. High blood sugar caused by gestational diabetes can also lead to exceptionally large babies.

And if you had a big baby the first time around, watch out, because, on average, subsequent babies tend to be around 7 ounces bigger. This may be because the uterus is already primed to grow new blood vessels, meaning more nutrients get through to the baby in subsequent pregnancies, helping them to grow bigger and stronger.

. 17 .

Why do some women show more than others? And why do women show earlier on in second pregnancies?

Although no one seems to have studied this phenomenon, it's widely accepted that women on their second or third pregnancy tend to look a month "bigger" than first-timers at the equivalent stage and usually have to dig out their maternity jeans much sooner.

Normally, the abdominal muscles on either side of the body are held together by a strip of connective tissue, but during pregnancy, a hormone called relaxin weakens that tissue, and as the growing baby pushes against the abdominal muscles from the inside, they begin to separate.

Andrew Satin, professor of obstetrics at Johns Hopkins University, says that in his general experience, women with stronger abdominal muscles tend to show less, and their abdominal muscles are less likely to be pulled apart during pregnancy. Women with smaller body frames are also likely to look bigger compared to tall, broader women.

The most plausible explanation as to why second-time moms show sooner is that their abdominal muscles are already weakened and stretched from the first pregnancy, and so provide less resistance against the hungry baby growing inside them, adds Stephanie Prendergast, a physiotherapist who specializes in postnatal care at the Pelvic Health and Rehabilitation Center in San Francisco. "As a general rule, they also tend not to be in as good a shape as they were prior to the first baby, because they're already caring for a baby and don't have time to exercise as much," she says.

. 18 .
Does a woman's body shape permanently change after pregnancy?

As your bump grows bigger, you may notice that it isn't just your waistband that seems to be getting tighter. During the first six months of pregnancy, most healthy women can expect to gain an extra 8 pounds of fat, which will be deposited on mostly the hips and thighs as an energy reserve for breast-feeding.

The good news is that ultimately, your legs and butt may end up skinnier than they were before you got pregnant—although many women end up slightly heavier overall.

Unlike men, young women tend to pile 30 to 40 pounds of fat on their hips and legs during puberty, which often stubbornly refuses to shift, regardless of how much exercise they do. But during the last ten to twelve weeks of pregnancy, and certainly once the baby is born, some of these fat reserves begin to be mobilized. Well-nourished breast-feeding women lose around 1.7 pounds of fat per month, much of it from previously protected reserves on the hips and thighs.

William Lassek and Steve Gaulin at the University of California at Santa Barbara analyzed data from 16,635 American women and found that, although they tended to gain weight with each successive pregnancy, the women's hip and thigh circumferences decreased with every child they had. If they regained any weight after pregnancy, it tended to be deposited on their waists and upper bodies.

Lassek points out that fat mobilized from the hips and thighs provides a good source of an omega-3 fatty acid called DHA, which is critical for brain growth. "During the first year of life, the brain increases by almost one kilogram," he says (1 kilogram is 2.2 pounds). "Mobilized maternal fat may provide critical fatty acids and energy for brain growth."

Although many women are overweight, Western diets are often deficient in DHA (which is found in cold-water fish such as salmon). A well-rounded backside is therefore good for your baby's health and something to be embraced. And you can potentially look forward to a new wardrobe of short shorts and miniskirts once the fat melts away.

. 19 .
Can Jacuzzis and saunas really cause miscarriage?

Your growing baby is insulated from the outside world by a thick layer of fat and muscle, so any changes in outside temperature are going to take a while to filter through.

However, sitting in a hot tub or sauna for a long time will cause your body temperature to rise, and there is some evidence that if it stays over 101°F for a long time, particularly in the first trimester, this can increase the risk of miscarriage and birth defects. It's important to note that most studies suggesting links between hot tubs and birth defects or miscarriage haven't studied the relationship between the two directly but either looked at women who had prolonged bouts of fever during pregnancy (and these illnesses may also have influenced the outcome of the pregnancy) or conducted their research on animals. The most convincing human study found a rate of two to three neural-tube defects per thousand women among those who had been in a hot tub during the first trimester, compared to the normal rate of one defect per thousand women. However, this study didn't record how hot the water was or how long the women stayed in. Also, it asked women about their hot-tub use after their baby had already been diagnosed with a birth defect, so they may have been more likely to recall the experience than women with healthy babies.

If you do decide to use a hot tub when pregnant, the American College of Obstetricians and Gynecologists advises never letting your core body temperature go above 102.2°F. Since most hot tubs are around 104°F and it takes only ten to twenty minutes of sitting in a hot tub to raise your body temperature to this level, women are often told to limit their time in a hot tub or sauna to just ten minutes.

Of course, your body temperature will begin to drop as soon as you step outside the tub, and even nonpregnant women tend to exit the sauna or hot tub when they begin to feel uncomfortably hot—a good sign that your body temperature is rising.

Taking a warm bath during pregnancy is a different matter. The top half of your body is not usually immersed, and the water is not constantly being heated, so it takes longer for your body to heat up.

Rumors also circulate that bathing during pregnancy might increase your chances of an infection that could trigger miscarriage, from bacteria in the water making their way up the vagina and into the uterus. During pregnancy, however, a thick plug of mucus in the cervix effectively seals off the uterus from the outside world, making that scenario extremely unlikely. Some studies have hinted that it may be more of a problem once a woman's water has broken, although the evidence is weak (see 49: "Can I take a bath once my water has broken?").

. 20 .
Is it safe to have sex?

Normally, the vagina is linked to the uterus by a narrow tunnel through the cervix, which the sperm must navigate in order for a woman to become pregnant. However, sperm have a hard time getting through once a woman is pregnant, because a thick plug of mucus blocks the tunnel. This plug also seals off the uterus from the millions of bacteria living in the vagina, reducing the risk of any infection that could damage a growing baby. One of the first signs of labor is the release of this plug—known as the "show"—when a blob of thick, occasionally bloodstained mucus appears in your underwear.

Even if any semen did get through the mucus plug, the baby is encased in a tough pair of membranes called the amniotic sac, so it's extremely unlikely that any semen could ever reach the baby.

. 21 .
Why do so many human embryos miscarry before twelve weeks?

It's a statistic that haunts most women during the early weeks of pregnancy: As many as one in three pregnancies end in miscarriage in the first trimester. I spent the first months of both my pregnancies obsessively checking off the days until my twelve-week scan, convinced that when I got there, the sonographer would find a blank space where my baby was supposed to be. I have friends who have been through the trauma of successive miscarriages, and the overriding question they ask is whether there is anything they could have done differently. According to the latest thinking on the main causes of miscarriage, the answer is almost definitely no.

"I don't believe that jogging around the block, or having sex, or having a glass of wine, or eating unpasteurized cheese is going to knock off an embryo that's destined to be successful," says Lesley Regan, an expert in recurrent miscarriage at Imperial College, London. "It's usually just coincidental."

A major cause of human miscarriage is that an egg that contains an abnormal number of chromosomes has been fertilized, also known as aneuploidy. Such embryos may grow for a while, but they often stop growing and abort during early pregnancy (sometimes before a woman even knows she is pregnant). Humans seem particularly prone to this problem compared with other mammals, though no one really understands why. For a woman between the ages of thirty and thirty-five, about 60 percent of human eggs are aneuploid, and this rises to over 90 percent for a woman in her early forties. "Over the age of thirty-five, the miscarriage rate goes up dramatically and the fertility rate goes down, so many, many pregnancies are lost," says Regan.

As well as helping to explain why so many pregnancies fail, this helps to explain why it can take so long to get pregnant in the first place, particularly as we age. Even among young healthy couples who diligently have sex several times around the day of ovulation, it can take months for the woman to become pregnant. It's not necessarily that she isn't conceiving but that huge numbers of embryos are lost before a pregnancy test would even detect their existence.

Some of the commonly cited statistics about miscarriage before twelve weeks can be misleading because they are heavily dependent on when you take a pregnancy test. Take the "one in three" figure. This seems to come from a study that confirmed pregnancy at the earliest point possible (before most commercial pregnancy tests would show a positive result). It found that 22 percent of pregnancies ended before they would have been detected using a normal pregnancy test, and 31 percent of pregnancies were lost overall. In other words, it isn't relevant to the everyday woman who has just found out that she's pregnant after doing a test she bought at the pharmacy, because if the pregnancy has progressed far enough for it to be detected using a home test, the risk of miscarriage has already dropped significantly.

Slightly more accurate is the "one in five" figure provided by the UK's Royal College of Obstetricians and Gynaecologists. This refers to women who have done a pregnancy test and got a positive result. Although the rate may still feel worryingly high for most couples, it's worth bearing in mind that it refers to the general population rather than individuals, and some women are at greater risk of having a miscarriage than others. Age is a factor, as is having had a previous miscarriage, while certain medical conditions such as diabetes or thyroid disease can also increase your risk.

Over twenty years ago, Regan conducted a study to assess the risk of miscarriage among different groups of women. Once pregnancy was suspected, the women came in for an ultrasound scan, and these scans were then repeated every two weeks until week twelve. Overall, she found that 12 percent of the women miscarried, but for first-time pregnancies, and for women whose last pregnancy resulted in a healthy baby, the risk of miscarriage was more like 5 percent—while for women who had carried several healthy babies to term, the risk dropped to 4 percent.

Others were at greater risk of miscarriage. Among women whose last pregnancy had miscarried, the risk was 19 percent, while for women who had experienced several miscarriages, their risk of miscarrying in this pregnancy was 25 percent (although that still meant that 75 percent of them had healthy babies).

The message is pretty clear: If this is your first baby, or your previous pregnancies have been healthy and you are showing no symptoms of miscarriage (such as pain or bleeding), then there is a far higher chance that you will carry a healthy baby to term than suffer the tragedy of miscarriage. That risk also drops the later in pregnancy you progress.

Exercise

. 22 .
Is it safe to exercise during pregnancy?

Many women stop doing vigorous exercise such as jogging during pregnancy for fear that it will increase their risk of miscarriage or damage their baby in some other way.

Although at least one large study has suggested that high-intensity exercise for more than seven hours a week increases the rate of miscarriage, most of the data was collected after miscarriages had occurred, so women may have recalled their exercise levels differently or been more motivated to take part in the study in the first place. Other studies have hinted that strenuous exercise might temporarily divert blood away from the fetus, meaning it gets less oxygen.

On the other hand, there is also some preliminary evidence that exercise during pregnancy results in leaner babies with advanced brain development and lower heart rates—something that could have lifelong benefits for health.

Current guidelines in the U.S., UK, and other countries advise women that they can continue exercising at a level of intensity similar to before they got pregnant, unless they have certain medical conditions, such as heart disease, or they have been told their pregnancy is at risk, because of prolonged bleeding, for example. When the Cochrane Collaboration explored the issue in 2009, it concluded that there is insufficient evidence to say whether exercise is good or bad for the baby, although aerobic exercise two to three times a week would improve or maintain the mother's fitness level.

However, emerging evidence suggests that even strenuous exercise during pregnancy isn't harmful, provided that the exercise program is tailored to the mother's level of fitness. Andrew Satin at Johns Hopkins School of Medicine asked heavily pregnant women to walk or run on a treadmill until they reached their maximal exertion threshold (the point where they can go no further). All the while, the movement and heart rate of the baby were monitored for any problems or signs of distress, as was blood flow to the uterus and amniotic fluid levels.

Even in women who didn't exercise before pregnancy, no impact on the baby's health was observed. "Contrary to what we believed in the past, it is even okay for women who have previously been inactive to initiate exercise during pregnancy," says Satin.

Although you might imagine that jogging would cause a baby to be flung around in all directions, Satin was surprised to see little change in the baby's position. "The uterus moves up and down, and the baby moves with it, but we really didn't observe radical changes of position at all," he says.

Above all, women who choose to exercise while pregnant should listen to their own bodies and slow down or stop if they feel light-headed or unwell. Pregnancy is not a good time to push through the pain and keep going. Satin also advises drinking plenty of water to prevent dehydration, and to avoid any activity where you might fall or get hit, such as skiing, horseback riding, mountain biking, or martial arts. This is particularly important as the baby grows bigger and ceases to be protected by the bones of the pelvis (typically, after around twelve weeks of pregnancy), when a serious knock could cause the placenta to become detached from the uterine wall, putting both mother and baby at risk.

. 23 .
What stomach exercises can I do when pregnant?

Although you should probably avoid lying on your back for prolonged periods during the latter half of pregnancy, this doesn't mean you can't exercise your abdominal muscles. In fact, it's important to maintain strong abdominal muscles during pregnancy, because these help support the pelvic floor and maintain your posture, which can be thrown off balance by that ever-bulging bump.

Exercises that should be avoided are full sit-ups, abdominal crunches, and those that involve twisting over to one side. The central abdominal muscles begin to pull apart during late pregnancy, and these exercises can widen that gap even farther. (For tips on how to close the gap once your baby is born, see 71: "Can other countries (for example, France) teach us anything about getting back into shape after birth?")

One exercise that is okay during mid- to late pregnancy is the transversus exercise, which can be done in any position. Place both hands below your belly button, take a deep breath in, and then pull the abdomen and belly button in toward the spine on the out breath. Hold this contraction for up to ten seconds, breathing normally, and repeat up to ten times.

Exercises such as the plank are also fine. Lying on your front, pull your belly button in tight and push up off the floor with your hands or elbows shoulder-width apart and your leg muscles engaged. You can also do a side plank, where your weight is supported on one hand or elbow and your feet. Both of these exercises can be made easier by bending your knees and using them to support your weight rather than your feet.

Pelvic tilts can help to strengthen the back as well as the abdominal muscles. Lie on your back with your knees bent and your feet resting on the floor, then tighten and pull in the abdominal and buttock muscles while pressing the small of your back into the floor.

. 24 .
Will lying on my back harm my baby?

During late pregnancy, the added weight of the baby, the amniotic fluid, and the placenta can start to compress the large vein that carries blood from the lower half of the body back to the heart, pooling blood in the legs. Rather than harming the baby, the most likely impact is that it will make the mother feel light-headed or dizzy, so she will want to turn over—although if she continues to lie on her back, that might ultimately reduce the amount of blood reaching the baby. However, I could find no published evidence to prove that lying on your back harms your baby.

Even in nonpregnant women, there is a slight decrease in the amount of blood the heart pumps when you lie on your back, compared with when you lie on your left side. One recent study that compared heart function in pregnant and nonpregnant women found a further drop once women reached around twenty weeks in their pregnancy, so this seems a sensible time to start to avoid lying flat on your back for prolonged periods.

Because this vein is on the right side of the body, lying on your right side can have a similar effect to being on your back. This may be why many women say they feel more comfortable lying on their left side as their pregnancy progresses.

"I think the key word here is 'prolonged,'" says Linda Szymanski, a professor of obstetrics at Johns Hopkins School of Medicine. Spending a couple of minutes on your back or right side is unlikely to cause any harm, but if you feel dizzy or light-headed, roll onto your left side.

. 25 .
Do pelvic-floor exercises actually work?

Here's a reason to start clenching those pelvic-floor muscles: They can boost your sex life. Your pelvic-floor muscles wrap around the inside of your pelvis, supporting and helping to control your bladder, vagina, and rectum. Midwives are constantly nagging pregnant women to do their pelvic-floor exercises—I still have red stickers dotted around my house to remind me to squeeze while watching television or brushing my teeth. These exercises can stave off the risk of developing urinary and fecal incontinence, which, sadly, affect a large number of women (at least temporarily) after birth. Up to 38 percent of women have some degree of urinary incontinence in the two to three months after birth, often a small amount of leakage when they laugh or sneeze, and up to 6 percent find it difficult to control their bowels. A recent review concluded that women who do pelvic-floor exercises during pregnancy are 56 percent less likely to develop urinary incontinence during late pregnancy and in the six months after birth than those who don't.

What fewer people know is that if you carry on doing these exercises after childbirth, it could improve your sex life. In a recent study conducted in Turkey, a group of seventy-five women who had given birth four months previously were divided into two groups, and half of them were taught how to exercise their pelvic-floor muscles. They started off contracting them for three seconds, followed by a three-second rest, then for two seconds ten times a day for fifteen days, after which they progressed to holding the longer contraction for five seconds, and eventually ten, and increasing the number of workouts to fifteen times a day.

By month seven, women who had been exercising their pelvic-floor muscles found it easier to become sexually aroused, were better lubricated, had more intense orgasms, and were more sexually satisfied than women who hadn't done the exercises. The pelvic-floor muscles are responsible for the rhythmical contractions of female orgasm, but they can also influence how well women respond to sexual contact, by affecting the location of the inner section of the clitoris, for example (see 71: "Can other countries (for example, France) teach us anything about getting back into shape after birth?"). Unfortunately, the evidence suggests that pelvic-floor exercises are unlikely to help you have an easier birth or reduce the risk of tearing. Given the other benefits, they seem worth the effort.

. 26 .
How do I know if I'm doing my pelvic-floor exercises properly?

Sometimes women think that they are clenching their pelvic-floor muscles when they're clenching other muscles, such as those of the buttocks. One way to check is to lie naked on your back in front of a mirror so that you can see the entrance to your vagina and anus. First, breathe in and relax your muscles, then start to squeeze from the back passage and up toward the muscles you would be using if you were trying to stop the flow of urine. You should see the anus contract, the area of tissue between the vagina and anus start to lift, and the entrance to the vagina start to close. "It should be a nice slow upward and inward movement," says Maria Elliott of SimplyWomensHealth in London, who specializes in pre- and postnatal physiotherapy. If you don't see this, it suggests that you're not tightening the correct muscles, so you should either try again or speak to a health professional.

Another tip is to use your breath to strengthen the force of pelvic-floor-muscle contractions. "You will get a much better pelvic-floor contraction on the out breath," says Elliott. "Long-term, the pelvic-floor muscles work with the abdominal muscles and diaphragm like a muscular cylinder. Doing squeezes down there is okay, but ultimately, the pelvic floor needs to start working as a team with those other muscles to get coordinated activation." Most hospitals recommend doing five sets of longer contractions and five to ten sets of short contractions five times a day, but the precise pattern varies. Elliott suggests cutting back on some and replacing them with some long, slow, breath-controlled contractions. To do this, take a deep breath into your rib cage and, as you breathe out, first pull in the pelvic-floor muscles and then zip in the belly button as if you are trying to squeeze into a tight pair of jeans. Relax as you breathe in, then repeat as you breathe out. Elliott recommends doing twelve of these out-breath contractions three times a day, ideally while lying on your side in bed or on the sofa, as soon as possible after having had your baby. Constipation and heavy lifting during the first eight weeks can cause prolapse, a dangerous condition in which the uterus begins to fall into the vagina.

Even if you don't remember to exercise your pelvic-floor muscles every day, the important thing is that you're doing some exercises rather than none. So get squeezing!

Baby on the Brain

. 27 .
Does pregnancy make women forgetful?

Losing track of what you were saying halfway through a sentence? Walking upstairs only to forget what you went there for in the first place? Many women claim to become more forgetful during pregnancy, though evidence for the existence of "momnesia," or pregnancy-related forgetfulness, is mixed. Some studies have shown that pregnant women score worse on tasks involving memory storage and retrieval, while others have found no correlation between pregnancy and forgetfulness.

One possibility is that women report being more forgetful because we expect pregnancy to scramble our brains so are more aware of any lapses in memory. However, brain scans have also shown that women's brains shrink during the final months of pregnancy and don't return to their previous size until around six months after birth—possibly because of the effects of hormones, or because the fetus is poaching nutrients for itself. This at least provides some evidence of tangible changes to the brain. On the other hand, we don't know if the shrinking has any effect on brainpower, or if it affects all areas of the brain equally. Experiments in rats have shown that the brain's memory center, the hippocampus, grows new neurons during pregnancy, so even if there is a short-term lapse in memory, there may be other, long-term benefits.

Even in the studies that have found evidence for momnesia, not all types of memory are affected equally. In one of the largest studies to date, 254 pregnant women were asked to do a series of memory tests that were repeated twelve to fourteen weeks after the birth. The tests were carried out on forty-eight nonpregnant women. Women in late pregnancy and new moms fared worse than nonpregnant women when it came to memorizing pairs of words (verbal memory). But working memory (or the ability to manipulate information already stored in the brain) and the ability to recognize faces were unaffected. Also, not all women were affected equally.

It's possible that what pregnant women lose in memory, they make up for in other areas. "The changes that are occurring may make you a better mother," says Laura Glynn at the University of California at Irvine, who led the study. Estrogen, in particular, aids the development of maternal instinct and nurturing, and high levels during pregnancy have been linked to increased feelings of attachment to children after birth.

In rats, at least, pregnancy and motherhood seem to trigger improvements in navigation skills and memory for places, which might make female rats better at foraging for food. Meanwhile, researchers at the University of Bristol, UK, have found that women's sensitivity to facial expressions showing fear, anger, and disgust increase during pregnancy, perhaps training them to become hyper-vigilant to threats once their children are born.

As pregnancy wears on, women seem to become less fazed by stressful situations. A classic way of testing stress in the laboratory is the Trier Social Stress Test—essentially, a mock job interview during which your body language and levels of key hormones are monitored. A study of 150 pregnant women found that the more advanced they were in their pregnancies, the less stressful they found the test. Women in late pregnancy also had lower blood pressure, slower heart rate, and less of an increase in cortisol during the test than women at twenty-one weeks of pregnancy and nonpregnant women.

We still don't know whether any of these changes are permanent, and what other beneficial changes might occur to the brain during pregnancy. "It is possible that when faced with different tasks related to the care of offspring, such as multitasking, performance under stress, or sensitivity to infant cues, mothers' performance might be enhanced," says Glynn.

. 28 .
Is stress during pregnancy bad for my baby?

If you believe what you read in the newspapers, stress during pregnancy triples your risk of miscarriage, doubles your risk of stillbirth, gives your child schizophrenia, asthma, and attention deficit hyperactivity disorder (ADHD), inhibits your child's emotional growth, and lowers your child's IQ. Indeed, if you type "stress" and "pregnancy" into Google, you get close to 77 million results. It's enough to raise your blood pressure just thinking about it.

But before you pack in your job and lie in bed for the rest of your pregnancy, you should know that many of these studies relied either on animal studies or on women recalling how stressed they were rather than measuring their stress directly; or they involved events far more stressful than taking a crowded bus to work or pulling an all-nighter to meet a deadline. The timing of the stressor and how you react to it seem to be important factors.

There are known mechanisms by which psychological stress could damage an unborn child. One possibility is that women who are stressed are more likely to smoke, drink alcohol, eat badly, or not make it to prenatal checkups. But stress also prompts the release of several hormones, including cortisol, which helps your body cope with stress by providing a quick energy boost and heightened awareness. Usually, cortisol production is quickly shut off, but in very stressful circumstances, such as losing a relative or living through an event such as a war or an earthquake, this doesn't happen, leading to chronically high levels. Studies in animals have shown that high cortisol levels can shrink areas of a baby's brain involved in memory storage, as well as trigger miscarriage and preterm birth. Cortisol and related hormones can also decrease blood flow to the uterus, and dampen the immune system, leaving you more prone to infection.

However, stressing animals in a lab isn't the same as understanding how stress affects pregnant women. Human studies have produced far more mixed results, with some suggesting there is an effect and others showing no effect. One of the biggest problems is defining what stress is, but there are issues of timing as well. There is some evidence that women who lived through a big earthquake during pregnancy may have given birth prematurely more frequently than other women—but only in those women who experienced the earthquake during their first trimester. These women also described the event as more stressful than women in their second and third trimesters. Similarly, pregnant women living near the World Trade Center in New York on September 11, 2001, had slightly more preterm births than women living elsewhere, but only if they were in the first trimester at the time of the attacks. However, among women who experienced the Chernobyl disaster in Ukraine, there was no increased risk of preterm labor.

One way to get around this problem is to do something called a meta-analysis, which involves combining the results of numerous independent studies to see what they say on average. When Heather Littleton at East Carolina University did this with thirty-five studies on stress and pregnancy, she found that babies born to stressed mothers were slightly more likely to have a low birth weight or to be underweight in the weeks after birth, but the effect was tiny. "On average, these studies are finding that stress only accounts for one percent or less of the variability in individuals' outcomes, such as the weight of their babies," says Littleton. The remaining 99 percent is down to other things, such as genetics and social or lifestyle factors.

Another way of investigating how stress affects unborn babies is to study it directly. Janet DiPietro and her colleagues at Johns Hopkins University examined 112 healthy pregnant women living in the U.S. three times during their third trimester. They asked the women about their stress levels and recorded how much the baby was moving. They also examined the babies two weeks after birth. The babies of stressed moms seemed to be more active and, after birth, more irritable, but they also scored higher on a brain-maturation test and had better control of their body movements.

Since cortisol is known to play a role in normal brain maturation, it's possible that moderate, short-lived stress during pregnancy might boost this process and even be good for babies. DiPietro says that pregnant women should take it easy but not worry about moderate levels of everyday stress. "Relaxation is good during pregnancy—if you like to relax. But there is no evidence that everyday stress has any adverse effects on the baby's development," she says.

. 29 .
Can men get pregnancy symptoms, too?

Nausea, heartburn, abdominal pain . . . If you thought it was just women who suffer these symptoms during pregnancy, think again. Although it's not officially recognized as a disease or mental illness, somewhere between 11 and 50 percent of men are thought to experience symptoms of couvade syndrome, or sympathetic pregnancy. The most common symptoms include loss of appetite, toothache, nausea, sickness, and anxiety. Symptoms tend to peak in the third month of pregnancy, when many women are suffering the evils of morning sickness, then diminish in the second trimester, only to rise again during the final month.

The term "couvade" derives from the French verb *couver*, meaning to hatch or sit on eggs. People have put forward various theories for why couvade syndrome might exist, including the man seeing the unborn child as a rival for his partner's affection and therefore unconsciously trying to attract her attention, or it being a physical manifestation of the identity crisis triggered by the prospect of becoming a father.

Although very little research has been done on the causes of couvade syndrome, those studies that do exist suggest that men are more likely to suffer symptoms if they are highly involved in their partner's pregnancy and in preparing for the birth.

If couvade syndrome sounds to you like just another form of male hypochondria, there may yet be a physical source of the symptoms. One study found higher levels of the hormone prolactin and lower levels of testosterone in men reporting more than two couvade symptoms, such as fatigue, altered appetite, and weight gain, compared to men with no symptoms—although just how these hormonal changes might trigger pregnancy-like symptoms in men remains unclear.

Regardless of whether you buy in to the existence of couvade syndrome, there is a pregnancy-related illness that men do suffer from and which should be taken seriously. Postnatal depression is estimated to affect between 4 and 25 percent of men in the two months following the birth of a child, although its onset may be more gradual than in women.

Having a partner who is experiencing postnatal depression is the greatest risk factor in men, and just as maternal postnatal depression can impact the baby's emotional development, paternal depression has a similar effect.

. 30 .
Why do women go into nesting overdrive in the final weeks of pregnancy?

I spent the final days of my first pregnancy baking, painting the nursery walls, sorting and re-sorting my daughter's new clothes, not to mention sewing my first (and only) patchwork quilt to go in her crib. In my second pregnancy, I dismantled a secondhand double stroller and spent hours obsessively scrubbing the fabric parts to get them clean. It is said that women go into nesting overdrive in the final weeks of pregnancy, and hormonal changes may help to explain this. For most of a pregnancy, progesterone dominates over estrogen, but as the birth approaches, estrogen levels begin to rise, and studies have found that women experiencing a greater shift in estrogen report more feelings of attachment and well-being once their babies are born. High levels of the hormones oxytocin and prolactin prompt the onset of maternal behaviors, such as becoming hyper-responsive to anything baby-related, raising the pitch of your voice, and becoming generally more touchy-feely.

Studies of rats hint at how these hormones might affect the brain on a physical level. As birth approaches, several structures at the front of the brain that have been linked to mothering seem to grow in size. These include brain areas associated with addiction and reward, the processing of emotions, and empathy. Pregnancy also triggers the growth of new brain cells in areas associated with learning and memory, and in rats, at least, these changes seem to be permanent: boosting their memory for places and their foraging abilities, and making them less anxious in the face of challenges. This pattern of new cell growth is reinforced with each subsequent pregnancy. Assuming the same changes take place in humans, this means that the more kids you have, the more "mommy-fied" your brain will become as you shift from a life that centered around your own needs to one where others take precedence. Most moms agree that they never stop worrying about their child or children, no matter how old they get. I feel as if I'm more vigilant and aware of threats now that I'm a parent, and I become claustrophobic if I take my children into a busy store. The hormone we know most about is oxytocin, sometimes referred to as the "cuddle chemical" but more accurately described as a hormone involved in forming relationships with others. Levels of oxytocin are boosted in pregnant women and remain high once the baby is born and possibly for much longer (although no one has measured it beyond three years). Those same brain areas associated with emotional processing and reward are highly responsive to oxytocin, and elevated levels are related to more sensitive parenting in both moms and dads.

Although these hormonal shifts may prepare women to feel maternal once their child is born, the system is reinforced by experience. Oxytocin is released in response to cuddling and spending time with your baby, so the more you play with your child, the more your natural parenting instinct will be activated.

Breast-feeding also triggers the release of oxytocin. A recent study that compared oxytocin levels in breast-feeding mothers with women who were bottle-feeding their infants found higher levels in the breast-feeding women. When the same women were played a recording of either their own or a different infant crying, the researchers noticed greater activation in the brains of breast-feeding moms in response to their baby's cry. Although this doesn't necessarily mean that breast-feeding makes you a more sensitive mother, it does show how important oxytocin is in driving maternal behavior.

. 31 .
Are some women naturally more maternal than others?

If you scan the brain of a woman three weeks after she has given birth, you will see greater activation of the areas involved in emotional processing, reward, and addiction—precisely the same areas that are stimulated when you fall in love. As different as maternal and romantic love may seem, on a physical level, having a baby is almost identical to meeting the partner of your dreams.

Obsession is one example. An area of the brain, the striatum, which is linked to obsessive behavior, is activated when we fall in love and when we have a baby. If you've been in love, you will remember those heady early days when you're constantly replaying conversations in your mind and checking to see if your lover has called. Moms and dads show symptoms of obsessive-compulsive behavior in the early days after their child's birth, such as ritually checking whether the baby is breathing or is warm enough.

However, not all women react to the birth of their baby in exactly the same way. Ruth Feldman at Bar-Ilan University in Ramat-Gan, Israel, has found that new mothers can be divided into two categories based on brain activity. She focused on two brain networks, one that links an area associated with emotional processing to social areas associated with empathy and reading cues given by babies, and the other linking an area associated with reward and addiction to the same social areas.

Although mothers showed activity in both brain networks when interacting with their babies, some showed more activity in the reward and addiction network, while others showed more activity in the emotional-processing network. The first group of women essentially became addicted to their babies, though they were also extremely in tune with their needs. Feldman calls them "synchronous mothers." "Their main feeling is reward, energy, and enjoyment," she says.

For women showing greater activity in the emotional-processing areas, "the overwhelming feeling is anxiety, looking for harm, and a sense of 'I need to protect my infant,'" Feldman says. This style of mothering could have evolutionary advantages preparing a child to be vigilant of surroundings and less trusting, for example. The payoff is being less aware of the infant's nonverbal signals, such as expressing tiredness. Feldman calls these women "intrusive mothers."

Although less common, there was a third category of women who showed little activity in either network in response to their babies. These women were suffering from varying degrees of postnatal depression.

It's interesting that the children of these mothers showed differences in behavior at the age of three. "They behaved towards their best friends in the same way as their parents behaved towards them when they were infants," says Feldman. The children of synchronous mothers were more engaged with a friend's needs and better at sharing, while the children of intrusive moms were more fidgety and less able to tolerate tension. Meanwhile, children whose mothers had suffered from postnatal depression were more withdrawn and their social skills less developed.

As well as demonstrating the importance of recognizing and treating postnatal depression, this study suggests that women shouldn't necessarily expect to react in the same way to becoming a mom. Feldman also emphasizes that these instinctive behaviors can be changed with practice. For example, intrusive moms can learn to be more sensitive to signals, such as their baby turning away from them when it would like a rest. "When you see that, just wait patiently for the child to look at you again," Feldman says.

. 32 .
Do men change when they become dads?

Men often get bad press when it comes to fatherhood. For centuries, they have been groomed to believe that their biological role is to provide for the family rather than to play any active part in a child's upbringing. However, several recent studies have challenged this, suggesting that men also experience biological changes when they become fathers and that these can make them happier, more engaged dads—if they allow themselves to be.

As well as researching how mothers' brains change in response to childbirth, Feldman has measured levels of the hormone prolactin in men during the later stages of their partner's pregnancy. This hormone is best known for its role in triggering breast-feeding, but Feldman has found that male prolactin levels also increase as birth approaches. What's more, men with higher levels of prolactin seem to be more alert and responsive to their infant's cries once the child is born.

In a separate study, Feldman measured prolactin levels in forty-three first-time dads when their babies were six months old. She found that men with the highest levels of this hormone were more likely to engage with their child, encouraging it to explore and interact with new toys. Men's prolactin levels also shoot up when they hear their baby cry. But prolactin isn't the only hormonal change affecting new dads. Levels of testosterone drop, which may make fathers less aggressive and more attentive to their family's needs. At least one study has found that men with higher testosterone levels are less likely to give their children attention, while another study found that fathers with lower testosterone expressed more sympathy and a greater need to respond when they heard their baby cry. Falling testosterone may discourage men from looking elsewhere for sex while their wives are too busy breast-feeding to satisfy their needs.

Expectant fathers see increased levels of the stress hormone cortisol in the three weeks before birth, while new dads often experience a surge of the female sex hormone estrogen when their babies are born. Animal studies suggest that this triggers nurturing behavior in males.

Finally, Feldman has found that levels of the "cuddle chemical" oxytocin increase in new dads; this, too, seems to relate to paternal behavior. Dads with higher levels of oxytocin played with their children more often and seemed more attached to them than those with less of the hormone.

Unlike women, for whom oxytocin levels automatically rise throughout pregnancy and as a result of breast-feeding, oxytocin production in men seems to be more hands-on. In a separate study, Feldman found that fathers' oxytocin levels were boosted in response to playing and interacting with their children. In other words, when it comes to parenting, men reap what they sow. Probably the more fathers engage with their kids, the more their paternal instinct will kick in, producing happier, more nurturing dads.

The Developing Baby

. 33 .
When does a baby become conscious?

Throughout my own pregnancies, I've pondered the question of consciousness. Can a fetus make sense of its environment, and does it have a sense of identity? Can it think, dream, or feel pain? And does the emergence of these senses happen suddenly, like turning on a light switch, or is it more of a gradual process?

These are difficult questions to answer, not least because we've yet to come up with a proper definition of what consciousness is in adults, let alone in unborn babies who have no way of describing their experiences to us.

A key moment is when the peripheral nervous system (all the nerves relaying movement and sensations from limbs and tissues outside the brain) joins up with the cerebral cortex (the brain region responsible for higher thought processes, such as memory, awareness, attention, and language). This connection, which occurs at around twenty-five weeks, is a vital link between the outside world and the higher brain. Without it, it is impossible to be aware of your surroundings or to make sense of them, says Hugo Langercrantz, an expert on fetal consciousness at the Karolinska Institute in Stockholm, Sweden. This includes becoming conscious of pain—although it is clear that fetuses react to and move away from painful stimuli at much earlier stages of development.

So what has been running through the baby's brain before this point? By the end of the first trimester, when your baby no longer looks like a fleshy tadpole but is starting to look vaguely human, its brain circuitry is roughly equivalent to that of an earthworm or a marine snail, says David Edelman, a consciousness researcher at the Neurosciences Institute in La Jolla, California. Obviously, human brains are programmed to develop far beyond this, but twelve weeks after conception, the fetus has gotten only as far as building the circuits that allow it to respond to its environment by reflex, without any higher involvement from the brain.

By around seventeen or eighteen weeks, the nerves from the rest of the body begin to connect to the brain, bringing the baby's state of consciousness roughly in line with that of a reptile such as a snake. A reptile undoubtedly responds to its external environment, tracking down a mouse by sight and smell, for example, but most scientists don't think reptiles engage in higher thought processes, such as abstract reasoning, since they don't possess a cerebral cortex (the outermost, folded layers of the brain). This is a moot point, because neither do some birds such as ravens and parrots possess a cerebral cortex, yet they appear to possess some degree of language and an awareness of others.

At nineteen weeks, human embryos will withdraw from painful stimuli such as being poked with a needle. By twenty-three weeks, they release stress hormones such as cortisol, noradrenaline, and a natural painkiller called beta-endorphin in response to a needle prick—even though higher brain regions aren't yet involved in processing these responses. If unborn babies do feel pain at this stage, it's unlikely to be the type of pain we experience as adults, but it may be pain nonetheless. It's a bit like trying to put ourselves in the shoes of an injured animal—it's impossible, as our brains are wired differently.

At twenty-five weeks, that all-important connection between the cerebral cortex and the rest of the body is made, enabling human-like reasoning. However, even now it would be foolish to try to ascribe adult-like consciousness to a fetus. None of us can remember what it was like in the womb, and one reason may be that we didn't have the words or experience to make sense of the various sensations feeding into our brains. Many experts now believe that consciousness isn't an all-or-nothing phenomenon but a gradual turning up of the dimmer switch, which continues throughout early childhood.

In addition, unborn babies are kept relatively sedated in the womb through a combination of low oxygen levels and anesthetic-like chemicals produced by the placenta. Fetuses show cycles of sleep and wakefulness, and though there is some evidence that they can learn, only at birth do they fully wake up for the first time.

. 34 .
Does a wriggly bump equal a boisterous baby?

Just seven weeks into pregnancy, the developing baby makes its first movements. These start slowly, with gentle back bends, but by sixteen weeks the fetus will be capable of virtually the full range of movements that a newborn baby is capable of—more so, because it is not constrained by gravity. A sixteen-week-old fetus can hiccup, make breathing movements, yawn, touch its hand to its face, kick its legs, suck, swallow, and move its eyes.

Despite all this, expectant mothers rarely start to feel any movements before eighteen weeks of pregnancy and often much later. Some women describe it as a lurching motion, like being on a roller coaster, while others say it feels like a gentle popping. Rest assured, your baby's movements will only get stronger as time wears on, and some babies are particularly keen on making their presence felt.

During the second half of pregnancy, the baby changes position approximately once a minute and is active around 30 percent of the time. However, women perceive only around a tenth of their baby's movements, because the impact is buffered by the sac of amniotic fluid in which the baby floats. At twenty weeks, the baby takes up about half of the available space in the uterus, so it has considerable room in which to kick, punch, and spin around. By the end of the pregnancy, the baby takes up around 90 percent of the available space—even though the uterus has stretched significantly—so it is considerably more restricted in its movements.

When I was about twenty-three weeks pregnant with my first child, Matilda, I took part in a study that involved lying in an MRI scanner while a group of researchers from Imperial College, London, took live video recordings of her movements. When they played them back to me, I was astounded to see her kung-fu-kicking the inside of my belly, crouching and jumping, when all I had felt was the odd pop. She was even making pincer movements with her thumb and forefinger: something she didn't do again until she was around seven months of age. When she was slightly older, I was constantly pummeled by her kicks, particularly in the early evening, after I had eaten. Now a spirited toddler, Matilda is one of the most active (and exhausting) children I know.

So it's intriguing to hear of several studies suggesting a correlation between a baby's activity in the womb and temperament once it is born. Back in 2002, Janet DiPietro and her colleagues at Johns Hopkins University monitored the heart rate and body movements of fifty-two fetuses at twenty-four, thirty, and thirty-six weeks of pregnancy, then examined the babies at one and two years of age.

They found that babies who were more active in the womb seemed to be less distressed at age one when they were frustrated or restrained by their parents, and at age two were more interested in interacting with toys and strangers. There was also a difference between boys and girls. Boys that were particularly energetic at thirty-six weeks of pregnancy went on to become more active children, while the opposite was true for girls.

In a separate study, Ian St. James-Roberts and Praveen Menon-Johansson at the Institute of Education in London asked twenty women who were thirty-seven weeks pregnant to log their baby's movements for an hour every morning and evening for three days. After birth, the baby's sleeping, feeding, and crying patterns were recorded at one, six, and twelve weeks of age.

Although the unborn babies tended to produce the strongest kicks in the evening, these movements didn't really match up with the baby's activity levels after birth. What did match up were the more subtle movements that mothers could detect, particularly those occurring in the morning. Babies who moved a lot were more prone to crying, while those who were less active tended to be more peaceful.

As a general rule, the later in pregnancy you study it, the more an unborn baby's temperament seems to match up with its older self. But even very early in pregnancy, there may be a hint of what's to come. Shimon Degani and his colleagues at the Bnai Zion Medical Center in Haifa, Israel, used ultrasound to study the activity of twenty-two pairs of twins between eleven and fourteen weeks of pregnancy and found that the more active twin tended to be the more difficult, unpredictable, inflexible, and active after birth.

. 35 .
Can a baby detect its mother's mood?

How a mother is feeling during pregnancy can also affect her baby's movements. Many readers will be familiar with the opening scene of *The Sound of Music,* in which Julie Andrews skips gaily through alpine meadows belting her heart out. Kazuyuki Shinohara and colleagues at Nagasaki University in Japan showed this uplifting scene to ten women during the last trimester of pregnancy while at the same time using ultrasound to count the number of arm, leg, and body movements their babies made. The women also watched a tear-jerking clip from the classic boxing movie *The Champ*. During both movies the women wore earphones, so their babies couldn't hear the sound track.

When the women watched the happy film, their babies waved their arms, while during the sad movie, their movements decreased. Although this study included only a small number of women, this does hint that a baby can detect its mother's moods. One way this might occur is through hormones such as adrenaline, which are released during times of stress or sadness and can redirect blood flow away from the uterus, which the baby might pick up on. Janet DiPietro is also studying how fetuses respond to their mother's emotional state. I met her when I was twenty-six weeks pregnant with my first baby, and she allowed me to take part in a study she was running. She has a theory that the bond between mother and baby forms long before birth, and one aspect of this involves the baby tuning in to its mother's emotions. I lay down, and a monitor was wrapped around my belly to detect my baby's heart rate and movements. Electrodes were stuck to my fingers and chest to pick up my heart rate and other physical responses that might be generated, and I was shown a series of videos about giving birth.

First I watched a happy film in which new mothers talked about their birth stories. I felt warm and excited about my own approaching labor and the baby I would soon meet. Then the film changed, showing graphic scenes of women experiencing difficult births and C-sections, which made me want to look away from the screen.

What's interesting is how my unborn baby seemed to react to these scenes. When we looked at the trace of her movements, there was a clear change in her behavior during the gory video: First she stopped moving, as if paying attention to what was going on in my body; then she started wriggling all over the place. DiPietro is still analyzing the results of the study to see if her theory holds up, but an earlier study did find a connection between a baby's response to its mother's emotions before birth and what the baby was like once it was born. The baby's heart rate generally slowed and its movement was reduced when its mother watched the birth videos, although the heart rates of many babies shot up during the graphic birth scene if the mothers became agitated by it. Those babies who were the most in tune with their moms' emotions seemed to be more irritable six weeks after birth. Curiously, the relationship may work both ways, with fetal movements having an unconscious effect on the mother as well as possibly training her to become alert to the child's needs and fall into line with its activity patterns so as to be ready for when it is born. DiPietro has found that every time a fetus moves, its mother's heart beats slightly faster and her fight-or-flight response is stimulated, even if she isn't conscious of the baby's movements. Although more research is needed to understand the significance of this finding, DiPietro has some ideas. Until recently, the assumption was that the relationship between mom and baby was just one-way, but the research suggests that it's a bidirectional relationship, she says. "The mom's body affects the fetus, but the fetus also affects the mom. I think it's preparing women to pay attention to their infants."

. 36 .
What do babies learn during their time in the womb?

A baby is wrenched bleary-eyed and sticky from its mother's body, a blank slate upon which its life and experiences will be etched. If this is your perception of the moment of birth, think again. A newborn baby has already clocked up a raft of sensations and experiences from its time in the womb.

Two months before a baby is born, it is already behaving pretty much as it will once it enters the wider world. Although it spends around 90 percent of its time asleep, that sleep is divided up into REM sleep, when its eyes dart back and forth under its eyelids, and non-REM sleep. When its eyes are open, it can see (as some light occasionally filters into the womb, bathing it in an orange glow), and for several months, it has been able to hear as well. Taste and touch are not neglected, as the unborn baby is treated to a cocktail of flavors from its mom's diet and spends its waking hours exploring its own body and the inner walls of its mother's soft, warm uterus.

Along with these senses comes the ability to remember. Take sounds. From around twenty-two to twenty-four weeks of pregnancy, a baby's ears have developed enough for it to hear noises from the outside world, and the baby may sometimes "jump" in response to a particularly loud noise. Although many of these sounds will be muffled by the mother's tissue and amniotic fluid, frequencies of around 125 to 250 hertz—the fundamental frequency of the human voice—remain relatively clear, which means that an unborn baby can tune in to its mom's voice, as well as to the sound of other noises in the environment. Several studies have inserted microphones into the uteruses of pregnant women, so we know that a baby's world is far from silent. There is the ongoing thump of the mother's heartbeat and the "swoosh" of blood pumping through her arteries. There are the gurgles of her digestive system and the distorted sounds of the outside world. The mother's own voice is the loudest, as it is conducted through her bones and down into her uterus. Studies have also found that the baby's heart slows when its mother talks, suggesting that it knows her voice and is comforted by it.

This suggests that unborn babies can remember voices. Several types of memory have been demonstrated in fetuses, from basic habituation (where you learn to filter out irrelevant noises like the ongoing hum of a dishwasher) to classical conditioning (where you learn to associate an object or action with a particular outcome). Pavlov's dogs, the most famous example of classical conditioning, were trained to associate a ringing bell with being fed, so eventually, the mere sound of a bell ringing made them salivate in anticipation of what was to come.

The earliest study to demonstrate that fetuses could learn was undertaken in 1925 by a German pediatrician named Albrecht Peiper. He noticed that a fetus would jump if a car horn was sounded close to its mother's belly during late pregnancy; after a few beeps, it no longer seemed to notice—a form of habituation. More recent studies have shown that a baby can habituate itself to sounds from around twenty-two to twenty-four weeks of pregnancy.

Unborn babies can learn to associate a piece of music with relaxation, which might prove a practical way of calming your baby after birth. In one study, pregnant women were conditioned to relax when they heard a twelve-second burst of music. After birth, those babies who had listened to the music during pregnancy stopped crying, opened their eyes, and made fewer jerky movements when they heard the same piece of music. Such associations are thought to form after around thirty-two weeks of pregnancy.

In addition, unborn babies seem to remember everyday sounds without being conditioned to respond in a certain way. In one famous experiment, Peter Hepper of Queen's University in Belfast studied a group of women who regularly watched the Australian soap opera *Neighbors* during their pregnancies to see if their babies could learn the theme tune. When they were played the tune several days after birth, they stopped moving and became more alert, and their heart rates dropped, suggesting that they remembered it, while babies who had never heard the tune showed no response. None of the babies responded to unfamiliar tunes. Hepper did this experiment with thirty-week-old fetuses and thirty-seven-week-old fetuses, but only the thirty-seven-week-olds could remember the tune after birth. What's more, if the theme tune was played to these babies twenty-one days after birth, their memory of it apparently had been lost, suggesting that fetal memories may be fairly short-lived.

Researchers at Maastricht University have also been testing the length of time fetuses hold on to memories. They found that if they placed a vibrating wand on a pregnant belly, this generally prompted the baby inside to kick—at least the first time they felt it. However, babies quickly got used to the vibrations and began to ignore them. The researchers then tested how long it took babies to start responding to the vibrations again, assuming that this would be a measure of their memory of the experience. In thirty-week-old fetuses, it took just ten minutes, but by thirty-four weeks, babies seemed to remember the vibrations for at least four weeks.

Although most experts agree that any memories formed in the uterus are likely to be fairly basic, and many animal fetuses have shown similar learning abilities, this doesn't mean that fetal learning isn't important. One theory is that these memories help to ease the transition between the womb and the outside world by teaching babies what sounds are "safe," so they aren't alarmed by everyday noises such as the doorbell or the television after birth.

All of this suggests that there may be ways of making your unborn baby's introduction to the wider world smooth. Read it a nursery rhyme, sing it a song, and continue doing the same thing once it is born. If nothing else, it may help bring you closer to the little person you're going to meet in just a matter of weeks.

. 37 .
Will playing Mozart to my bump make my baby more intelligent?

For some ambitious parents, it's never too early to start trying to boost their baby's academic performance. Several studies have suggested that playing classical music to infants can boost their intelligence; the phenomenon has been dubbed "the Mozart Effect." This has led to the development of several "antenatal universities," usually programs of music or natural sounds designed to be played to babies during the final weeks of pregnancy to kick-start their brain development.

This idea started in the 1980s when a researcher called Donald Shetler played classical music to the abdomens of sixteen pregnant women at the Eastman School of Music in Rochester, New York, and noted that this seemed to be associated with the early development of "highly organized and remarkably articulate speech" once the children were born.

Since then, several studies have hinted that classical music can boost spatial reasoning, or the ability to imagine objects and reason with them (which is important in fields such as architecture and engineering), when played to young children.

In 1998, a study was published showing that rats exposed to different types of music while in the uterus and during the first sixty days of life showed different levels of performance when put into a maze. Those that had listened to Mozart completed the maze more quickly and with fewer errors than rats that had listened to music by modern composer Philip Glass, white noise, or silence.

Whether the same applies to humans is less clear. Human fetuses do show changes in heart rate and movement in response to both music and the human voice. They also seem to remember music or sounds they have been exposed to during their mother's pregnancy (see 36: "What do babies learn during their time in the womb?"). Evidence that classical music has any lasting effect on human babies remains weak, however. "There are many claims but as yet no work has been published of peer-reviewed scientific standard to demonstrate they actually have an effect," says Peter Hepper.

That's not to say that playing music to your unborn baby is harmful. It may relax you, and your baby will probably respond to that. It may also ease your baby's transition into the outside world by providing it with something familiar. And even if Mozart doesn't make your baby brainier, it may have other benefits. In one study, playing Mozart to preterm infants on two consecutive days seemed to boost their weight gain, seemingly by relaxing them and reducing the amount of energy they burned.

. 38 .
Will my baby look like Mom or Dad?

Most parents believe that their child is the most gorgeous being on the planet, no matter what anyone else thinks. The chances are you'll also rate your partner as pretty attractive. But maybe there are facial features you secretly hope your child isn't landed with, and this probably applies to your own features as well. It might be a father's prominent nose or your thin lips that you'd prefer your baby didn't inherit.

We all inherit some genes from our mother and some from our father, but several things happen on the way to making a new baby to ensure that he or she is unique. The first happens before the baby is even conceived. Most cells in our bodies contain forty-six chromosomes (twenty-three from our mother and twenty-three from our father); egg and sperm cells are exceptions, containing just twenty-three chromosomes in total.

When eggs and sperm are made, every chromosome you inherited from your mother matches up with the equivalent chromosome from your father, and they shuffle their genetic information before being divided between two new cells. This means that some of your mom's genes will end up next to your dad's genes on the same chromosome, and each new egg and sperm cell will have lost around half of your mom's and dad's genes.

That's not the only way genetic variation can occur. Once an egg is fertilized, mutations can creep into the embryo's DNA as its cells divide, and although the maternal and paternal copies of most of the twenty-thousand-odd genes the baby inherits will be equally active, in a small number of cases, the mother's or father's copy will be switched off. One example of this is the genes that control the formation of the placenta, which is guided largely by the father's genes.

Although most people agree that children tend to take after their parents, it isn't easy to pinpoint exactly how physical characteristics, such as the size of your nose or the shape of your teeth, are inherited. Rather than being controlled by a single gene, as some diseases are, physical traits are usually the result of lots of different genes working together, often combined with the effects of the physical environment.

Even eye color isn't as simple as it once seemed. People used to believe that variations of a single gene determined your eye color, with brown eyes being dominant over blue and green. This is still broadly true, but we now know that there are about sixteen genes that can influence eye color (some more than others). People used to think that it was impossible for two blue-eyed parents to have a child with brown eyes, and if they did, then the mother must have been sleeping with someone else. In fact, because of the complex interplay of all these genes, up to 25 percent of children with blue-eyed parents may end up with brown eyes, depending on the genes their parents possess.

Hair color is similarly complex, with one exception: red hair. A gene called MCR1 seems to be the key player in deciding whether or not a child has red hair, and the flame-haired variant is recessive. This means that if a child has one copy of the red-hair variant and one copy of the non-red-hair variant, he will not have red hair (although he will be a carrier, so his children might have red hair—and carriers often have freckles). The only guarantee of a flame-haired child would be if both parents have red hair. But a blond and a black-haired parent could have a 25 percent chance of a red-haired child if both of them are carriers of a red variant.

The inheritance of facial characteristics such as high cheekbones or full lips is less well studied, but several research groups have tried. In one Icelandic study, researchers compared the bone structures of 363 children's faces with those of their parents when the children were six and sixteen. The pattern was by no means clear-cut, but boys were more likely to resemble their mothers than their fathers, while daughters were influenced by both parents. An earlier Japanese study also noted that sons were less likely to inherit their father's features—particularly their nose shape—while daughters were influenced by both parents. Although the development of bones and teeth is likely to be a complex interplay between many different genes and environmental factors, these studies hint that several important genes determining bone structure may lie on the X chromosome, which means that sons would inherit only their mother's copies.

. 39 .
Do unborn babies dream?

Unborn babies spend an enormous amount of their time asleep, but at around thirty weeks, this sleep starts to become organized into more adult-like patterns, with four distinct states, from deep sleep to awake. However, there is a key difference: Both fetuses and newborns spend far more time in REM sleep than older children and adults, and this is the sleep state associated with dreaming.

Obviously, it's impossible to know what fetuses are dreaming about, and the sort of complex dreams that we experience in adulthood aren't thought to emerge until around five years of age. But unborn babies are immersed in a rich environment of touch, tastes, sounds, and movement, so it's quite possible that they are using their REM sleep to rehearse or fine-tune things they've learned during the day. "Given the fetus's senses are operating and it has the potential to learn, it could be dreaming about the day's experiences," says Peter Hepper.

REM sleep also seems to be important for the fetus. Certain drugs, including some antidepressants, will suppress REM sleep, and animal studies have suggested that disrupting REM sleep in fetuses results in increased anxiety, disturbed sleep and breathing, and abnormal brain signaling once they become adults. One explanation is that REM sleep may help to perfect the firing of brain cells, ensuring that they are in balance.

Another function of REM sleep might be to train the brain to "wake up." The transition between sleep and waking involves the coordination of several brain structures that are involved in controlling breathing and heart rate, so it is important that these "learn" to interact properly. REM sleep activates many of these brain structures, so it may be serving as a kind of rehearsal for when the baby has to make these transitions without the life-support system of its mother's blood and oxygen supply.

Weirdly enough, fetal "yawning" may play a similar role. Babies start to yawn from around eleven weeks and do so until birth. "Yawning appears to be not just a matter of opening one's mouth but a generalized stretching of muscles," says Olivier Walusinski, a physician based in Paris who has been investigating this phenomenon. Both fetuses and newborn babies yawn twice as frequently as adults, stretching their mouth muscles once or twice every hour. Yawning also seems to trigger the transition between periods of rest and activity, and as in REM sleep, many of the brain regions involved in waking seem to be stimulated by yawning.

. 40 .
Are babies more active at night?

Many mothers report that their bumps seem particularly prone to kicking at night. Researchers have also noticed this (see 34: "Does a wriggly bump equal a boisterous baby?"), although it may be that moms are simply more aware of these movements when they are horizontal because the blows are landing on different internal organs, or because they are not preoccupied with other activities.

As a general rule, unborn babies seem to synchronize with their mother's circadian rhythm or body clock, so they have some concept of night and day even if no light is reaching their eyes. This may be important in terms of teaching them to sleep and feel hungry at the correct time of day, in preparation for when they are born. Studies in rats have shown that disrupting a mother's body clock during pregnancy results in pups that feed at unusual times of the day. Babies born prematurely seem to have less well-developed circadian rhythms, and there is some evidence that their growth and sleep patterns are disturbed as a result. Several studies have found that preterm babies whose nurseries are kept dark at night sleep and feed better than those in nurseries where the lights are on constantly.

Although such studies are still in their infancy, there may be lessons that all of us can take away: If babies are born with a notion of night and day, we should do all we can to reinforce it by giving them plenty of natural light in the daytime and trying to avoid turning the lights on during night feeds. Women should also do their best to sleep at night and get outside during the daytime during late pregnancy (see 100: "How can I get my baby to sleep through the night?").

. 41 .
How do fingerprints develop?

A ten-week-old fetus reaches out and brushes against the soft lining of its mother's uterus, and as it does so, amniotic fluid eddies and swirls around the tiny digits of newly formed fingers and toes, which are already showing the first signs of fingerprints.

For centuries, palm readers have claimed that the lines and creases of the hands and fingers can be used to forecast a person's destiny. That may be closer to the mark than you might imagine, as mounting evidence suggests that fingerprints can provide lasting clues about life in the uterus and may even hint at future risk of disease.

Between the third and fourth months of pregnancy, a baby's delicate skin transforms from a translucent two-layered coating to the more robust and waxy three-layered skin that we have as adults. As this third layer of skin forms between the two existing layers, it becomes buckled, and ridges develop on the skin's surface. These are the beginnings of fingerprints.

Fingerprint patterns are loosely divided into whorls, loops, and arches, although there is a lot of variation within these groups. Early in development, raised swellings called volar pads appear on the surface of nascent fingers and toes, which are thought to give rise to blood and connective tissue. Between weeks ten and fifteen, these pads stop growing and are absorbed back into the fingertips; precisely when this happens seems to determine the fingerprint pattern you are left with. If the pads are still prominent when the third layer of skin begins to form, you get whorls; if they have almost disappeared, you get arches; and if it's somewhere in between, you get loops. These patterns are genetically determined to some extent, but even identical twins show differences in their fingerprints, so some other factor is also clearly at work.

Henry Khan at the U.S. Center for Disease Control and Prevention in Atlanta has been investigating how environmental conditions could influence fingerprint development. Fingerprints were taken from 658 Dutch people born between 1943 and 1947 (some of whom were fetuses at the time of a famine that struck the Netherlands between 1944 and 1945), and the number of ridges on the thumbs and little fingers were counted. Most people have more ridges on their thumbs than on their little fingers, but Khan found a greater difference among babies conceived during summer than those conceived during winter. When they looked at the fingerprints of those who had been fetuses during the famine, this difference couldn't be seen, suggesting that unusually harsh conditions had altered their fingerprint patterns.

In a separate study, Khan looked at whether differences in the number of ridges between thumb and little finger might identify people at higher risk of diabetes. He took fingerprints from 577 people and asked them to take a glucose tolerance test (an early marker of diabetes). As predicted, Khan found that people with normal glucose tolerance had smaller differences in their ridge counts than those with diabetes. Although it's not clear how a baby's environment could alter its fingerprint pattern, one suggestion is that the availability of nutrients and the presence of stress hormones might interfere in some way.

TWO

BIᴦTH

Get a Move On

42.
Who decides when it's time to come out?

Having a baby is probably the most visceral time of a woman's life. For nine months, we are buffeted by hormones that make us sick, tired, emotional, and occasionally forgetful. Our bellies swell; our breasts ache; we grow stretch marks and strange new patches of brown skin. Once the baby is born, it is usually placed, slippery and warm, on our chest, and a new tide of hormones overwhelms us, prompting our breasts to leak milk and sending us on another crashing roller coaster of emotional highs and lows. The aspect that I found hardest to deal with was the loss of control over my own body—and nowhere was this felt more acutely than in the timing of the actual event: birth.

For nine months, I diligently counted off the weeks, each one taking me a step closer to the day that had been circled heavily in my diary since my first doctor's appointment: the due date. The two weeks before and all dates after were a no-man's-land of uncertainty. Finally, I reached my due date, and hey presto, I was still pregnant. I felt like I was trapped in limbo—impatient and utterly powerless.

The trigger of birth remains one of the biggest mysteries of the human body. For years, people assumed that the baby came out when the mother's uterus could stretch no farther and deflated like an overblown balloon, pushing the baby with it. A later view was that labor started when the mother was no longer able to supply enough oxygen and nutrients to sustain the baby's growth, and the baby somehow triggered its own delivery. More recently, the focus has shifted, passing the reins of control to neither mother nor baby but to the gelatinous mass that has sustained the baby's growth over nine months: the placenta.

Two hormones control the contractions that thin the cervix and expel the baby from the uterus: oxytocin and prostaglandin. It is these hormones that are given if labor has to be induced artificially or speeded up if it isn't progressing fast enough. But what prompts a woman's body to start producing these hormones in the first place?

This is a complex puzzle that scientists have spent years trying to unpick. Simplified, one of the current leading theories goes like this. Since shortly after conception, a tiny clock has been ticking in the cells that become the placenta, and it grows steadily louder and louder until those ticks can no longer be ignored. The physical manifestation of the clock is a hormone called CRH, which is produced by the placenta throughout pregnancy in larger and larger amounts until it reaches a critical threshold and unleashes a cascade of hormones that ultimately triggers birth.

First the baby's brain releases two hormones, ACTH and DHEA, which prompt the placenta to start churning out large amounts of estrogen. This in turn initiates the production of prostaglandin and oxytocin, kick-starting the contractions of labor.

The idea of a placental clock is a nice one, but it doesn't explain everything. For example, what causes the cervix to soften and prompts your water to break? One idea is that the immune system is involved. As the baby matures, its lungs begin to produce a substance called surfactant, which stops their moist linings from sticking together. But surfactant also gets out of the lungs and into the amniotic fluid, where it rallies immune cells to the uterus. These immune cells then release chemicals that soften the cervix and weaken the membranes containing the baby and amniotic fluid, making them more vulnerable to bursting. The fact that premature labor is often associated with infection lends support to the involvement of the immune system, as infection also activates the immune system.

Regardless of how it starts, it's true to say that labor varies massively among women, as does their perception of the pain it causes. Some get stuck in the first stage of labor for days. Others whizz through and spend most of their labor in the second (pushing) stage. Still others are unable to give birth vaginally and require a C-section. Labor is nothing if not unpredictable. The best advice is to keep an open mind and be prepared for all possible scenarios.

. 43 .
Can my state of mind delay labor?

My first child, Matilda, was due on August 31—the last day of the UK school calendar—which would have made her the youngest in her grade. Although plenty of geniuses have been born in August, there is some evidence that children who are the oldest in their school year are at an academic advantage, so I couldn't help inwardly crossing my legs and hoping Matilda would hold on for an extra day (she was born a week overdue in the end, which is common for first babies; see 44: "Is it normal for pregnancies to run past their due date?").

It's widely assumed that women have no control over when they give birth, but a recent study has challenged this. Rebecca Levy and her colleagues at the Yale School of Public Health examined eleven years of U.S. birth records dating from 1996 to 2006, paying particular attention to the two-week periods surrounding Halloween and Valentine's Day. Regardless of the type of delivery, women were 5 percent more likely to give birth on Valentine's Day and 11.3 percent less likely to give birth on Halloween than in the two weeks surrounding these days.

As Halloween often carries negative connotations of death and evil, Levy suggests that women may subconsciously want to avoid having a baby on that day, while Valentine's Day, with its associations of cute cherubs and love, may elicit the opposite reaction, although she hasn't yet pinned down a biological mechanism by which positive or negative thoughts could trigger labor.

. 44 .
Is it normal for pregnancies to run past their due date?

For centuries, the accepted wisdom has been that pregnancy lasts for nine calendar months and that you can calculate your due date by adding seven to the date of your last period, then counting back three months. This calculation became known as Naegele's rule, after the nineteenth-century obstetrician Franz Naegele, who first published it in 1812.

It may seem ludicrous that a two-hundred-year-old calculation is still used to predict length of pregnancy. Indeed, many hospitals now use ultrasound to confirm the expected date of delivery based on a baby's size at around twelve weeks of pregnancy, which is considered more accurate. Studies that have compared ultrasound dating to Naegele's rule have found that, on average, Naegele's date is three days too early.

However, this, too, is an average. First-time moms generally have longer pregnancies than women expecting their second, third, or fourth child. One study of Caucasian women found that although 61 percent of existing moms were overdue according to Naegele's rule, they were only three days late on average (as ultrasound dating would predict). In contrast, the average first-time mom gave birth eight days later than Naegele would have predicted, and 81 percent were overdue.

Pregnancy length also varies according to racial background, with more South Asian and black women giving birth before thirty-nine weeks than white women. Their babies seem to be more developmentally advanced than those of white women born at the same stage.

All of this could have medical implications. Most obstetricians believe that remaining pregnant beyond forty-two weeks may put the mother's and the baby's health at risk, so they tend to induce labors that run seven to fourteen days past the expected due date. The main reason they give is the increased risk of stillbirth among babies born after forty-two weeks, which doubles from one per thousand pregnancies at forty-two weeks to two per thousand pregnancies at forty-three weeks. However, if the due dates are out, then women may be induced unnecessarily, which can carry risks of its own (see 47: "Will being induced mean I'm less likely to have a natural birth?"). In industrialized countries, rates of induction range between 10 and 25 percent of pregnancies, with around 22 percent of women in the U.S. being induced—although there is an ongoing debate about whether this number is too high.

. 45 .
Can curry or anything else help trigger labor?

Sex, curry, raspberry-leaf tea—there are a multitude of home remedies for kick-starting labor. By the time women reach the fortieth week of pregnancy, they're usually desperate to meet their baby and will try anything to get the process moving. A friend of mine resorted to hours of frantic nipple-tweaking, which left her with very sore breasts, but she went into labor that night. Heavily pregnant myself, I tried imitating my friend but got nothing to show for it but a minor twinge. Pushing my skepticism aside, I paid a Chinese therapist thirty pounds for a massage, and eight hours later, my contractions started. An effective therapy, or was it simply that I was already seven days overdue and labor was destined to start anyway?

Fortunately, we don't have to rely on anecdote to find out whether such home remedies really work, as a number of scientific studies have been done to evaluate them.

Raspberry-leaf tea
For centuries, herbalists have been using the leaves of the common red raspberry (*Rubus idaeus*) to prepare the uterus, and a recent survey of U.S.-based midwives found that 63 percent of them recommend it for inducing labor. However, in studies where raspberry-leaf extract has been given to animals or added to strips of uterine tissue, the results have been mixed: Some showed that it relaxed the muscle, others that it caused more coordinated contractions, while still others suggested that it increased the length of pregnancy.

Even if raspberry-leaf tea does affect the uterus, it's not clear how much of the stuff you'd have to drink for the active ingredients to work their magic. One small study, which compared women who took raspberry-leaf tablets twice a day from thirty-two weeks with women who didn't, found a very small reduction in the length of the second (pushing) stage of labor in the women who took the tablets, but the effect didn't reach statistical significance, meaning that it could have been down to chance.

Curry or castor oil

Disappointingly, there have been no studies to assess the value of curry in initiating labor (I would happily volunteer if there were). The theory is that the spice in curry irritates the bowels and triggers muscular contractions that send you rushing for the bathroom but may also spread to the womb and initiate labor.

Better studied is castor oil, which is thought to have a similar effect. Castor oil has been used to induce labor since ancient Egyptian times and was recommended by obstetricians in Western countries until the 1950s, when newer drugs such as Syntocinon (a synthetic form of oxytocin) became available. It is still used in many developing countries. Apparently, it's pretty unpleasant to drink and may make you sick, as it has the taste and texture of very thick cooking oil. In 2012, an Israeli group announced the results of a prospective, randomized, double-blind, placebo-controlled study (which is about as good as it gets) on whether drinking castor oil induced labor: It found that the odds of entering labor within twelve hours of drinking castor oil were three times higher than if you drank sunflower oil. Women also seemed to progress through the first stage of labor more quickly. Unfortunately, there were just eighty women in the study, so more research is needed. Whether curry is an effective substitute, we don't know, but it would probably have to be spicy enough to give you diarrhea—in which case you might prefer castor oil. The usual dose is four fluid ounces, which can be chased with orange juice, although it may be wise to speak to your doctor or midwife before trying it.

Pineapple

Pineapple contains an enzyme called bromelain, which could theoretically help to soften the cervix—although whether it would survive the harsh conditions of the digestive system and get into the blood in high enough amounts to have any effect seems unlikely. Tasty as it is, there is no scientific evidence to support the use of pineapple in inducing labor.

Nipple stimulation

Tweaking, massaging, or pumping the breasts all spark the release of oxytocin, one of the hormones that causes labor contractions. A review of six trials involving a total of 719 heavily pregnant women found that more than a third of women who stimulated their breasts were in labor within seventy-two hours, compared to just 6 percent of those who didn't. The amount of time the women spent tweaking their nipples or pumping their breasts varied from a total of one to three hours a day (with rests in between), and the women generally switched breasts every ten to fifteen minutes.

Although some doctors fear that nipple stimulation might overstimulate the uterus and potentially upset the baby, the review found no evidence of that (although its authors suggest avoiding nipple stimulation in high-risk pregnancies, just to be on the safe side). Nipple stimulation seemed to reduce the risk of excessive bleeding after birth, presumably because the extra oxytocin caused the woman's uterus to contract more strongly and close off the blood vessels feeding the placenta after birth. A shot of oxytocin is often offered to birthing women in order to achieve the same effect.

Sex

Although sex may be the last thing on your mind when you're about to give birth, many people will tell you that semen contains prostaglandins, which help to ripen the cervix. Possibly this rumor was started by men in a last-ditch effort to get some action before the baby arrives, but it seemed logical enough to warrant further investigation.

Swedish scientists recently asked twenty-eight heavily pregnant women either to have unprotected sex "with vaginal semen deposit" three nights in a row or to avoid sex completely. Because breast stimulation might have an independent effect, both groups were told that the nipples were absolute no-go areas. In this admittedly small study, sex didn't seem to do anything. There was no difference between the women in terms of the baby's position, the softness of the cervix, or the number of women who gave birth within the next three days. Having sex is unlikely to harm the baby, but it's also unlikely to hasten its birth.

Acupuncture

A handful of small trials have suggested that women receiving acupuncture are less likely to be medically induced, but because these women knew whether they were receiving genuine acupuncture, there may have been a placebo effect at work. Many other studies have found no effect.

Homeopathy

The Cochrane Collaboration recently reviewed two trials of homeopathy in inducing labor. One found that women taking a mixture of black cohosh (*Actea racemosa*), arnica, caulophyllum, pulsatilla, and gelsemium twice a day from thirty-six weeks of pregnancy spent an average 5.1 hours in labor, compared to 8.5 hours for those who took a placebo pill, and suffered fewer complications—although the authors of the review said the study was too small to draw any firm conclusions. The second study looked at women whose water had broken prematurely and found that those taking an hourly dose of caulophyllum took an average thirteen hours to begin regular contractions, compared to 13.4 hours in women taking no supplements—a small enough difference for it to be down to chance.

. 46 .
Does having a membrane sweep work?

If you sail past your due date, you might be offered something called a membrane sweep. It's not the most dignified or comfortable procedure, involving a doctor or midwife sticking her fingers into your cervix and trying to stretch it and (if she can reach that far) separate the membranes containing the baby from the top of the cervix. This supposedly releases prostaglandins that further soften and thin the cervix, hastening the onset of labor.

Just how successful your doctor will be depends on the state of your cervix when she carries out the sweep. At forty to forty-one weeks, some women will have started to dilate, while others may be experiencing contractions even though their cervix shows little sign of softening, and the doctor may struggle even to reach it.

Plenty of studies have investigated whether membrane sweeping works, with mixed results. For this reason, the Cochrane Collaboration tried to review as many studies as it could in an attempt to draw some firm conclusions about the procedure. Generally speaking, membrane sweeping does increase your chances of going into labor within forty-eight hours or giving birth within the next week if you are already overdue—although it's no guarantee. Eight women would need to have a membrane sweep in order for just one of them to avoid medical induction of labor, and it's hard to know if you'd be in the lucky minority. Having a membrane sweep at thirty-eight to forty weeks of pregnancy also slightly reduces the chances that you'll still be pregnant at forty weeks.

It's a fairly unpleasant procedure and may trigger bleeding and painful contractions that don't result in labor. In one of the studies reviewed, 70 percent of women reported significant discomfort, while a third reported significant pain. For this reason, the review's authors say the rationale for membrane sweeping healthy women who aren't overdue is questionable.

. 47 .
Will being induced mean I'm less likely to have a natural birth?

A woman sails through pregnancy healthy, happy, and excited about meeting her baby for the first time. As the due date passes, frustration and impatience can set in, but for women who remain stubbornly pregnant once they pass the forty-one-week barrier, a new terror awaits: the threat of induction.

Supporters of natural childbirth sometimes warn that being induced will make contractions more painful and difficult to cope with, which means that you're more likely to need an epidural, which in turn can make a C-section or instrumental delivery (involving forceps or a ventouse) more likely. What's more, because induction is a medical procedure, your baby's heart rate will need to be monitored continuously, which makes it harder to move around during labor or use a birthing pool.

The evidence suggests that many of these fears are overblown (see 66: "Does an epidural make a C-section more likely?"). Medical induction is usually recommended once women reach forty-one or forty-two weeks, and several drugs can be used. The first strategy is usually to give prostaglandins to help soften the cervix and make it easier to open. If this doesn't help, a plastic tube can be inserted into the back of the hand to provide a drip containing Syntocinon (an artificial version of the hormone oxytocin, which regulates contractions).

Some studies have indicated that women who are induced tend to request an epidural sooner than those entering labor naturally, which might suggest that the contractions are more difficult to cope with. It's also possible that because induction is generally carried out in a hospital ward under a doctor's supervision, women are simply more likely to be offered an epidural rather than being encouraged to use other methods of pain relief.

So what about the claim that being induced increases your risk of needing an emergency C-section? So widespread is this dogma that in 2009 the U.S. Agency for Healthcare Research and Quality (AHRQ), which produces guidance for doctors, decided to take a closer look. Although some studies have suggested that induction boosts the risk of having a C-section, they've tended to compare women who are induced to women who enter labor spontaneously. This might seem reasonable, except that most women who are induced are overdue, so it would be better to compare them with other overdue women who are simply waiting and monitoring the situation. These women may eventually enter labor spontaneously, or they may have to be induced—but watchful waiting can bring problems of its own, such as ending up with an excessively large baby who needs to be delivered by C-section anyway.

After reviewing seventy-six studies, the AHRQ found that women who were induced were 20 percent less likely to need a C-section than women who simply watched and waited. Their babies were also around 50 percent less likely to have meconium (poop) in their amniotic fluid, which is a sign of maturity and is more common in post-date babies but can increase the risk of breathing problems. Most of the studies analyzed looked at women at or beyond forty-one weeks of pregnancy. Before this, the risk of C-section appeared to be more or less equal in both groups of women. Two other large reviews published within the last ten years reached similar conclusions.

Women may fear that if being induced makes an epidural more likely, then it may boost the risk of an instrumental delivery (one involving forceps or a ventouse). A separate review of nineteen trials found a slightly increased risk of instrumental delivery among women who were thirty-seven to forty weeks pregnant when they were induced, but this disappeared when one looked at women who were forty-one to forty-two weeks pregnant. This is important because most women who worry about being induced will fall into the second category. Bear in mind that if your pregnancy is overdue and you aren't induced, then your baby will keep on growing and may be harder to push out when the time does arrive. A similar picture emerges if one looks at women who are offered a Syntocinon drip, since their labor slows or stalls. Overall, it seems to shorten labor and ultimately make women less likely to need a C-section or instrumental delivery.

The message I take away is that although being induced may quash your dreams of a home or midwife-led birth, if you're still pregnant two weeks past your due date, then it may be worth listening to the advice of your doctors. You can still hope for an otherwise uncomplicated natural vaginal delivery, and it may ultimately be safer for both you and the baby.

. 48 .
Will rocking on my hands and knees cause my baby to turn over?

By the end of pregnancy, 90 percent of babies are head down and two-thirds of them are facing their mother's spine, which is the optimum position for fitting through her pelvis. However, a stubborn few seem determined to face the other way around, which makes birth more painful, and a breech baby who remains head up will often need to be delivered by C-section.

Because the head is the heaviest part of the body, people may tell you to get down on your hands and knees and use gravity to turn a difficult baby. Unfortunately, there is little published evidence to suggest that this works. One recent review of three studies by the Cochrane Collaboration found that although getting on hands and knees for ten minutes a day caused a baby to rotate in the short term, it didn't stay that way for long. Several other studies suggest that, although babies may shift position according to what the mother is doing at the time—aligning their bodies with the mother's when she rests, for instance—they often revert to the original position or a different position afterward.

Women shouldn't give up on the hands-and-knees position entirely, though: The Cochrane review found that it was effective at relieving back pain during labor.

Midwives may also try using something called external cephalic version (ECV) to turn a breech baby, which involves prodding and pushing at your bump in order to encourage the baby to flip a somersault. Success rates for this technique range from 35 to 57 percent for women in their first pregnancy, and from 52 to 84 percent for existing mothers, so it seems worth a try.

. 49 .
Can I take a bath once my water has broken?

Relaxing in warm water is a great way of staving off early labor pains, but women are sometimes told that it is dangerous once water has broken because bacteria in the bathwater could be flushed into the uterus and infect the baby. This rumor seems related to a common distrust of water births, once considered dangerous because of fear of infection.

However, when Swiss researchers compared the risk of infection in mothers whose water had ruptured, they found no difference between those who took a warm bath and those who didn't.

Several studies looked at infection rates in women who choose to have water births and found no increased risk of infection in either mother or baby. Despite water becoming contaminated with feces during a water birth, some obstetricians believe that it may even help to protect newborns against subsequent diseases and allergies (see 54: "Are vaginal births really better than C-sections?").

The Big Push

. 50 .
Why do humans find it so difficult to give birth?

Watch a dog or a horse giving birth, and its babies just seem to slip out, with none of the pain and screaming associated with human labor. During my first pregnancy, I fell for a book that told me because animals have relatively pain-free births, women can have a similar experience if only they banish fear. Having gone through labor, I now think this theory does women a great injustice in implying that pain relief means you have somehow failed. Research highlights several reasons why humans don't give birth like animals—and none of them have anything to do with eliminating fear.

In the grand scheme of things, we humans have existed for only a wisp of time. Although the first mammals appeared a hundred million years ago, when dinosaurs still roamed the earth, our early ancestors began walking on two legs only around three million years ago. The transition from four legs to two required that the human pelvis became narrower, but since then, its size has remained pretty much unchanged, while the human brain has almost quadrupled in size. "Human labor is an uneasy compromise between our need to run and our need to think," says Philip Steer, professor of obstetrics at Chelsea and Westminster Hospital in London. "We're erect bipedal animals, but we have very big brains."

A sheep's or rat's uterus is paper-thin compared to that of a human, because a lamb or rat pup meets little resistance on its journey into the wider world. In contrast, the human uterus is a powerful muscle that can take hours to push the baby out.

Even some of our closest living relatives have an easier time of it than we do. Imagine a hard-boiled egg cut in half, with the yellow yolk surrounded by a thick rim of egg white. If a baby gorilla's head is the egg yolk, then the egg white is similar in proportion to the amount of space a baby gorilla's head has when it passes through its mother's pelvis. Although it has to push against muscle and soft tissue, there is no bony pelvis standing in its path.

Now imagine trying to squeeze a golf ball through an egg-shaped hole: It barely fits. That's how a human head looks in proportion to a human pelvis. All those brain areas we've developed that give us personality, and the ability to forward-plan and socialize, come at the expense of having to squeeze the head out at birth. We've adapted to some degree, as the bones of the human head will overlap when squeezed (which is why many babies born vaginally have "cone heads" to start with), but it's far from easy.

. 51 .
Why are human babies born so helpless?

The challenge of, effectively, squeezing a pinhead through the eye of a needle also helps to explain why human babies are born so helpless. Human pregnancies last an average of forty weeks, which is similar to those of chimpanzees or gorillas, but human babies are born premature by comparison. Besides not being able to walk until a year, a newborn human has a brain that is just a quarter of the adult size, compared to half the adult size for baby chimps and gorillas. This is probably so that the head remains small enough to fit through the birth canal. "The joke is that if humans were born as mature as chimpanzees, human pregnancy would have to last seventeen months," says Steer. "Think of the complaints we would get in the antenatal clinic then!"

In addition, human babies have to twist their way through the birth canal in order to get out, which means that they usually come out with their head facing their mother's bottom, unlike other apes, whose babies are born face-up. This may be why midwives exist in virtually every human society that has been studied. Although other apes see their baby's face emerge, can clear any mucus from its mouth and nostrils, and remove the umbilical cord from around its neck, it's simply not practical for humans to give birth on their own.

. 52 .
What's the biggest baby ever born?

According to *The Guinness Book of World Records,* the largest baby ever born was a boy weighing 23 pounds, 12 ounces, and measuring 30 inches in length. That's around three times the average weight of 7 pounds, 8 ounces, and 10 inches longer than average. The boy was born to a giantess named Anna Bates, who herself stood 7 feet 5.5 inches tall, in Seville, Ohio, on January 19, 1879. Sadly, the baby died eleven hours later.

The heaviest baby born to a normal-sized mother and father was a boy weighing 22 pounds, 8 ounces, who was born to Carmelina Fedele in Aversa, Italy, in September 1955. More recently, an Indonesian woman gave birth by C-section to a boy weighing 19 pounds, 3 ounces, in 2009. The mother was diabetic, so high sugar levels in her blood may have fueled the baby's growth.

The title for smallest baby goes to Amillia Sonja Taylor of Florida, who was born weighing just 10 ounces and survived, despite being born extremely premature—at twenty-one weeks and six days of gestation.

As for the largest number of children born to one woman, Fyodor Vassilet gave birth to sixty-nine children during her lifetime. Born in Russia in 1707, she experienced twenty-seven pregnancies, giving birth to sixteen sets of twins, seven sets of triplets, and four sets of quadruplets, before dying at the age of forty.

. 53 .
Is there any way to predict how long labor will last?

When I was expecting my first baby, I was told that I should look to my mother's experience of labor for an idea of how my own would progress. She said it took around nine hours from her first contraction to my slithering into the world. So when my own contractions started at one A.M. on a Monday morning, I diligently switched on my TENS machine and fully anticipated that I would have my baby in my arms by lunchtime.

Twenty-four hours later, I was in the hospital being told that, despite having contractions every three minutes for the past six hours (and my contractions having come every three minutes for the past six hours), my cervix had dilated only three centimeters and I was barely in "active labor." It wasn't until seven-thirty P.M. on Tuesday that my daughter finally burst into the world—some thirty-two and a half hours late by my original calculations.

The average length of labor for a first-time mom is somewhere between thirteen and seventeen hours and can be divided into three stages. The first stage is when the cervix is thinning and dilating to the point where it is open enough to let the baby's head through, which typically takes twelve to fourteen hours for a first-time mom (although this first stage can be subdivided into a latent phase, when contractions are occurring but the cervix isn't dilating, and an active phase, when it is steadily dilating). Next is the second or "pushing" stage, which typically takes one to two hours, followed by the third stage, which involves expelling the placenta and takes up to an hour. It is true that subsequent labors tend to be faster than the first—around six to eight hours for the first stage of labor and five to sixty minutes for the second stage.

Several things are known to influence how long or difficult a woman's labor will be. In terms of the first stage, women whose baby's head has not yet started pressing on the cervix (known as engagement) tend to have longer latent phases. Weirdly, this is also true of women who have had more than five babies, presumably because their uteruses are weaker and less able to push the baby against the cervix (although the second stage of labor tends to be much faster in these women). Obese moms also tend to have longer first stages of labor, although the reason for this is unclear.

More is known about the factors that can slow down the second (or pushing) stage of labor. An obvious one is the size of the baby, as bigger babies tend to take longer to push out and are more likely to get stuck. The size of your pelvis is important, but just because you have big hips doesn't necessarily mean you'll have an easier labor, because the shape matters, too. As a general rule, Afro-Caribbean women tend to have narrower birth canals and are more likely to have trouble delivering if their babies are overdue. This is offset by the fact that they also tend to have shorter pregnancies.

One common myth is that the size of your feet can be used to predict how easy your labor will be. Back in 1988, Scottish researchers examined the association between height, shoe size, and the outcome of labor in 563 first-time moms. They found no significant difference in women's shoe size and the rate of C-section, whether they had to be induced, or the length of labor, although the babies of women with larger feet tended to be slightly heavier. However, when it came to height, they found that women who were shorter than five-three were more likely to need a C-section because of difficulties with the baby's head fitting through the pelvis. Even so, 80 percent of women shorter than that managed to have a vaginal birth.

Another important factor is the position of the baby as it enters the birth canal, which can affect the chances of it getting stuck. Babies whose head is facing toward their mother's belly as they enter the birth canal are harder to squeeze out, as they will need to make more twists and turns during their journey.

Sadly, none of these factors is easy to control or even possible to predict on an individual basis. But there are some steps you can take to increase the chances of your own labor progressing smoothly. Several studies have suggested that women who eat normally in the twenty-four hours before labor and get a decent amount of rest and sleep are more likely to have short labors than those who are tired and hungry. So be sure to keep your energy levels up, drink plenty of water, and (if possible) sleep during the early stages of labor, as this extra energy should help when things get tougher.

. 54 .
Are vaginal births really better than C-sections?

The media has long lambasted women who opt to have a C-section rather than pushing their baby out the natural way. In the UK, they're labeled "too posh to push," the assumption being that women choose to have a C-section either for reasons of convenience or because they are too afraid to go through labor.

Not only are these assumptions insulting to the majority of women who have a C-section for perfectly valid reasons, they are also largely incorrect. Cesareans are on the rise in many countries, and currently, 31.8 percent of American women give birth by C-section (around a quarter in the UK), yet there's little evidence that more than a handful are doing it for nonmedical reasons. An audit of 32,082 C-sections performed in the UK found that just 7 percent were performed at the mother's request; of these, it's not clear how many involved women with underlying medical problems or those who previously gave birth by C-section. When women expecting their first baby were asked, just 3.3 percent expressed a preference for a C-section.

Even if large numbers of women aren't pushing to have a C-section, a growing number of doctors believe they should be allowed to choose one if they so desire. In 2011, the UK National Institute for Health and Clinical Excellence (NICE) published guidance stating that all women should have the right to a C-section, even if there is no medical need. The main justification is that, as technologies have improved, C-sections have become far safer—particularly if they are planned, rather than performed as an emergency procedure.

In America, women can choose to have a C-section, although the American College of Obstetricians and Gynecologists (ACOG) recommends a vaginal birth in the absence of any medical necessity. If women do opt for surgery, AGOG recommends that C-sections shouldn't be planned before week thirty-nine of pregnancy; they shouldn't be motivated by fears that effective pain medication isn't available; and they aren't recommended for women planning to have several children, as every C-section you have slightly increases the risk of complications in subsequent pregnancies.

There are many myths and misconceptions about the relative benefits of natural birth versus a C-section. Having experienced both types of birth, I can assure you that there are upsides and downsides to both, but let's take a look at the evidence:

A vaginal birth is harder on your sex life

Many pregnant women worry whether their sex life will return to normal after giving birth. It's no reassurance that up to 24 percent of obstetricians and 45.5 percent of urogynecologists say that they would choose a C-section for themselves or their partner. The main reason is the higher risk of incontinence associated with vaginal delivery, although nearly 60 percent add that sexual dysfunction is another reason. But remember: Obstetricians and urogynecologists tend to see only the complicated births and worst cases of birth trauma in their clinics. Just 4.4 percent of midwives say they would opt for a C-section—testimony that the majority of women deliver their babies without complication and recover well afterward.

In the short term, there's no denying that having a baby will probably put a dent in your sex life, regardless of how you give birth (see 72: "Is it normal to be turned off by sex after birth?"). Up to 86 percent of women report sexual problems in the first few months after giving birth, and this is more likely among women who need an instrumental delivery (involving forceps or a ventouse) or who tear during birth. Such women often report pain in the area between the vagina and back passage in the eight weeks after birth, and sex may be uncomfortable for up to a year. Even a relatively minor tear or an episiotomy (a deliberate cut to help get the baby out) can be expected to lower your libido and make sex a little uncomfortable in the first three months.

You might assume that a C-section would avoid any such sexual problems, but when it comes to comparing straightforward vaginal births with C-sections, the picture is less clear. Although vaginal births carry a slightly increased risk of damage to the pelvic-floor muscles and the nerves connecting the vaginal area, one large study that compared planned C-sections with uncomplicated vaginal deliveries found that 18 percent of women who had a C-section reported pain during sex in the first three months, compared with 10 percent of women who gave birth naturally. Having a C-section involves cutting through the walls of the abdomen and uterus, so it's fairly normal to experience some generalized pain in that area. However, if you have a

C-section, you are more likely to have resumed sexual activity a month after birth.

The good news is that, a year on, most women have recovered their sex lives, regardless of how they delivered their baby. When 524 Dutch women were interviewed a year after giving birth, the majority said that they were sexually satisfied, and this was unrelated to the method by which they gave birth.

Vaginal births increase the risk of incontinence

One of the biggest fears surrounding vaginal birth is that it will increase your risk of incontinence. It is true that rates of urinary incontinence are lower in women who have had a C-section, compared to a vaginal birth, although it's no guarantee. This is because much of the weakening of the pelvic-floor muscles associated with motherhood comes as a result of hormonal changes during the early months of pregnancy. Scarring from a C-section can also put pressure on the bladder, making stress incontinence (where you may leak some urine when you cough, sneeze, or exercise) more common.

Estimates of the risk vary according to when and how you ask the question, but when a Canadian group recently combined the results of eighteen studies, they found that in the three months to two years after birth, the risk of stress incontinence was 16 to 22 percent among women who had vaginal births, compared to 10 percent for women who delivered by C-section. This would mean that ten to fifteen C-sections would have to be performed in order to prevent one case of stress incontinence. When the most serious cases of incontinence were looked at, there was very little difference between the two groups.

It takes longer to recover after a C-section

Many women are told that having a C-section puts them at increased risk of infection, postnatal depression, future infertility, and a longer hospital stay. However, the UK's National Institute for Health and Clinical Excellence (NICE) recently reviewed the literature and concluded that for many of these claims, the evidence was of very low quality. When Joseph Wax at Maine Medical Center reviewed the evidence, he concluded that for planned C-sections, at least, women are no more likely to suffer complications than those having a vaginal birth. Any risks also have to be weighed against the fact that women who have had a C-section generally describe a better birthing experience both in the immediate aftermath of the birth and three months later.

C-sections are associated with a longer hospital stay, but not much longer: an average three to four days, compared with one to two days for a vaginal birth. And if a woman who has had a C-section hasn't suffered any complications and seems fit and healthy, NICE recommends sending her home after twenty-four hours—albeit with painkillers.

Although it may take slightly longer to get back to your pre-pregnancy activity levels after a C-section, some women who have natural deliveries take extra time to recover as well. When nearly a thousand American women were interviewed seven weeks after birth, 65 percent of those who had a vaginal birth reported no limitations in terms of running, lifting heavy objects, and doing strenuous sports, compared to 45 percent of women who had a C-section; 90 percent of those who had a vaginal birth reported no limitations when lifting or carrying bags of groceries, compared to 80 percent of those who had a C-section.

It's true that having a C-section constitutes major abdominal surgery and therefore increases the risk of complications such as infection, blood clots, or blood loss, but there are steps that can be taken to reduce these risks. There is now strong evidence that women should be offered antibiotics before surgery in order to reduce the risk of infection, and they should be monitored for signs of blood clots. Women should take good care of the wound, showering or bathing daily, gently drying the wound afterward, and being vigilant for any signs of infection, such as increased pain, and any discharge, redness, or signs of the wound pulling apart. The same applies to women who tear during a vaginal birth and are at risk of infection.

When Italian researchers compared rates of complications in women undergoing planned and emergency C-sections and vaginal births, they found little difference in terms of the risk of infection or serious blood loss between the groups—apart from women who needed an instrumental vaginal delivery and were at greater risk of a serious tear.

C-sections make it harder to bond with your baby
The seeds of this idea can be traced to a speech given by the French obstetrician Michel Odent in 2006, who warned that pre-labor C-sections can inter-

fere with the natural production of oxytocin, which helps create a loving bond between mother and baby. This does not apply to women who are already in labor and require an emergency C-section, since they usually have been exposed to plenty of oxytocin (which triggers contractions) before being rushed in for surgery. There is scant evidence to suggest that a lack of oxytocin during birth has any long-term effect on maternal bonding.

One study from 1986 found that women who delivered by C-section handled their babies less frequently a week after birth than mothers who delivered vaginally, but the authors admit that this may be because of tiredness and discomfort, and they didn't check to see how mom and baby interacted several weeks or months down the line.

Similarly, a study published in 2008 suggesting that C-section moms were less responsive to their baby's cries than moms who delivered vaginally drew its results from just twelve women, and it used brain imaging to look at how areas related to empathy and reward were activated, rather than measuring hormone levels or seeing how the mothers reacted to their babies in everyday life.

One thing we know about oxytocin is that it is produced throughout the latter stages of pregnancy and is released in response to breast-feeding and simply cuddling and handling your infant, so you should get plenty of it in the aftermath of birth. "Especially if the baby is breast-feeding, the mom's brain will produce oxytocin and promote bonding irrespective of whether she got synthetic oxytocin or had a C-section," says Paul Zak, an oxytocin expert at Claremont Graduate University in California and author of *The Moral Molecule*.

Although bonding is difficult to measure scientifically, some studies have at least hinted that early skin-to-skin contact can help the mother bond with her baby. For example, when the mothers of thirty-two babies who touched or licked the nipple within thirty minutes of birth were compared with those of twenty-five babies whose first contact with the breast was around eight hours after birth, the researchers noticed that women who had experienced early skin-to-skin contact spent more time with their babies, talked to them more during breast-feeding, and had lower levels of a stress hormone during breast-feeding over the next four days than mothers who initiated breast-feeding slightly later.

There are steps you can take to try to make a C-section feel less clinical and more like a "natural" birth, which may in turn help to promote bonding. In its latest guidelines, the UK's National Institute for Health and Clinical Excellence recommends that women undergoing a C-section should be allowed to listen to music in the operating room, dim the lights, request silence so their voice is the first the child hears—even have the screen lowered at the moment of birth so the mother can watch her baby being born. Assuming there are no complications, they should also be given early skin-to-skin contact if they want it, as this can boost the chances of successful breast-feeding.

C-sections make breast-feeding more difficult

A number of studies have found that women who deliver by C-section are less likely to breast-feed than those who have a natural birth. Why should this be? One clue lies in the fact that women who have had a C-section often take longer to put their baby to the breast than women who deliver vaginally. Mother and baby are usually monitored for several hours following a cesarean birth, and in many hospitals this takes place in separate rooms, which means that women don't get the chance to breast-feed and bond with their baby right away.

Italian researchers recently compared breast-feeding patterns between women who delivered vaginally, by planned C-section, and by emergency C-section. Upon discharge from the hospital, 88 percent of women who had a vaginal birth were breast-feeding exclusively, compared to 73 to 74 percent of women who had a C-section. When the researchers examined how long it took for the baby to be offered its first breast-feed, they found it took ten to thirteen hours for those babies delivered by C-section, compared to three hours for babies delivered vaginally. Many researchers believe that such delays interfere with a baby's natural impulse to seek out the breast and suckle in the immediate aftermath of birth, before they get too sleepy. It could also interfere with the onset of milk production in the mother's body, making it harder for breast-feeding to get started.

However, hospitals are waking up to the idea that women who have had a C-section might want to enjoy immediate skin-to-skin contact with their baby (see 83: "Does skin-to-skin contact really soothe my baby?"). This is particularly true of planned C-sections and when women remain awake during the operation. In a recent pilot study at San Francisco General Hospital, the proportion of women getting skin-to-skin contact with their babies within ninety minutes of a C-section was increased from 20 percent to 68 percent thanks to an awareness drive among medical teams, which in turn boosted the rate of breast-feeding. Among babies who didn't experience skin-to-skin contact within the first ninety minutes of life, 74 percent needed additional formula milk in the next few days, while only 30 percent of those who got early skin-to-skin contact needed extra milk. "Skin-to-skin contact has historically been difficult to implement after cesarean birth due to common hospital procedures," says Kristina Hung, who led the study. "However, it is definitely something a woman can request on a birth plan, and it's something I would personally insist upon."

Women who have had a C-section may need extra help lifting and positioning the baby during the early days. Many breast-feeding experts recommend either lying on your side to breast-feed, or using a football hold, in which the baby is tucked under your arm with its legs dangling behind you in order to protect the wound. Women can also breast-feed in a reclined position, with the baby lying on top of them. Babies born by C-section are sometimes sleepier or less physically developed (if born prematurely), but with the right support, there's no reason they can't be breast-fed.

Babies born by C-section are less healthy

There are situations where babies born by C-section are almost certainly healthier. For example, if a baby is breech, its chances of dying or suffering serious injury during birth are around 5 percent if delivered vaginally, compared to 1.6 percent if it is delivered by C-section. However, babies born by C-section are at a slightly increased risk of breathing problems in the immediate aftermath of birth—although this risk drops sharply if the C-section is performed after thirty-nine weeks of pregnancy, when the lungs are more mature. Babies born by C-section are also marginally more likely to need resuscitating after birth, while babies born vaginally have a slightly increased risk of rare brain bleeds. Overall, there is no difference in short-term survival rates between babies born by C-section and those delivered naturally.

What about longer-term health? A number of studies have suggested that babies born by C-section are at greater risk of asthma and allergy when they get older. When a British group recently combined the results of twenty-three such studies, they concluded that C-section increased a child's risk of asthma by around 20 percent. This means that if nine out of a hundred children in the general population develop asthma, then approximately eleven in a hundred children born by C-section will become asthmatic. A separate review of twenty-six studies reached a similar conclusion about the risk of hay fever in babies born by C-section and found a 30 percent increase in the risk of food allergy.

This doesn't necessarily mean that C-sections cause conditions such as asthma. For example, premature babies and those with very low birth weight are also thought to be at increased risk of asthma, and these babies are often delivered by C-section. Breast-feeding is thought to afford some protection against asthma and allergy, and fewer moms who deliver by C-section tend to breast-feed.

There is one reason to think that babies delivered vaginally might be at a slight advantage: Natural birth is a messy business, and a newborn usually swallows a hefty dose of the bacteria that become smeared across its face. But this rarely causes illness, because the baby has already received antibodies against many of the thousands of bugs dwelling in the mother's body. These bacteria then go on to colonize the baby's own gut and help protect against infection and possibly allergic disease.

By contrast, a baby born by C-section never receives this initial inoculation by its mom's bacteria. Instead, the first bugs it encounters may come from the hands of a doctor or the towel in which it is swaddled. Such babies have been shown to have different gut flora than babies born vaginally, and there are some hints that this may leave them more vulnerable to asthma or allergies.

There may yet be a solution to this problem, though it's not for the squeamish: Some obstetricians have suggested taking a swab from the mother's vagina immediately after birth and rubbing it over the baby's mouth. This is probably best done only after consultation with your doctor!

. 55 .
Are home births riskier than hospital births?

In 2010, a study by Joseph Wax and colleagues at the Maine Medical Center in the U.S. generated headlines on both sides of the Atlantic with its finding that, although women who give birth at home suffer fewer complications, for some, the risk of the baby dying is tripled.

Even in the scientific journal where it was published, the study led to a flurry of angry letters from other researchers who disputed the conclusions. Wax responded by pointing out that in low-risk women who are cared for by highly trained midwives, planned home births actually reduce infant deaths. In other words, home births are safe so long as the right women are having them and they receive care from properly trained individuals. Unfortunately, the reputation of women who choose to have home births as being irresponsible mothers has largely stuck.

Currently, around one in two hundred women has a home birth in the U.S., compared with one in fifty in the UK. One reason for the disparity is that the American College of Obstetricians and Gynecologists remains concerned about home births, citing a lack of good-quality evidence to prove their safety, whereas both the UK's Royal College of Midwives (RCM) and the Royal College of Obstetricians and Gynaecologists (RCOG) support home birth for women with uncomplicated pregnancies.

Wax's 2010 study is one of the largest to tackle the issue of home birth, so it's worth taking a closer look at its conclusions. The study was actually a review, pulling together the results of twelve separate studies and analyzing a total of 342,056 planned home births and 207,551 planned hospital births within the U.S., the UK, Canada, Australia, and several European countries.

As you might expect, home births were associated with fewer medical interventions, including epidurals, electronic heart rate monitoring of the baby, C-sections, instrumental deliveries, and episiotomies, as many of these things are difficult to do at home. Even so, mothers who had home births experienced fewer infections, tears, and serious bleeds, compared to mothers who delivered in the hospital. This doesn't necessarily mean home births are better for women: The study included existing mothers, and if they had experienced complications during their first birth, they may have chosen a hospital birth this time around; women expecting large babies (who are more likely to tear) probably would have opted for a hospital delivery as well. Similarly, when it came to the babies born at home, these were less likely to be premature, of low birth weight, in need of additional help breathing than those born in hospital; many such babies would be considered high-risk and would need to be delivered in the hospital.

What about that tripling of the death rate that many newspapers picked up on? If you looked at death rates around the time of birth, there was little difference between babies born at home and in the hospital, which suggests it wasn't down to babies failing to be resuscitated or anything like that. The problem crept in if you looked at death rates in the twenty-eight days following birth. The risk was still small, 32 deaths for every 16,500 home births, compared to 32 deaths for every 33,302 hospital births. However, not all of the studies that Wax analyzed recorded this "neonatal death rate," and because the numbers are so small, it's difficult to say with certainty just how great the risk is. What's more, when Wax excluded those home births assisted by people other than certified midwives, there was no increase in the death rate between planned home and hospital births. The babies were just as safe, regardless of where they were born.

Of course, not all women are the same, and you might expect that some would be better suited to home birth than others. A separate study, published in 2011, supports this idea. Called the Birthplace study, it followed 64,538 English women who planned to give birth either at home, in a midwife-led unit or in a hospital maternity ward. It confirmed that, overall, the risk of something terrible happening to the baby is small—there were just over 4.3 reports of death or birth injury per 1,000 births.

If you looked at women giving birth for the first time, however, the risk of these adverse outcomes was significantly higher if they chose to give birth at home—there were 9.3 adverse outcomes per 1,000 births, compared to 5.3 when babies were delivered in hospital. What's more, 45 percent of first-time moms who'd planned a home birth were transferred to the hospital either during or shortly after birth.

It's a different story for women who already had a child. For them, the risks to the baby were similar, and just 12 percent needed to be transferred to the hospital.

Ultimately, no one really knows if home births are any riskier than hospital births, because the necessary studies haven't yet been done. This means you should be wary of well-meaning friends, relatives, and strangers who tell you that one is more dangerous than the other.

There are several factors you may wish to consider:

- Somewhere between 9 and 37 percent of women having a home birth will need to be transferred to a hospital during labor. The most common reasons include labor progressing too slowly or the woman needing additional pain relief, such as an epidural—and women are more likely to be transferred if it is their first baby. In more serious cases, women may be transferred because of heavy bleeding, concerns about the baby's welfare, or because the baby needs emergency care once it is born, and in these circumstances, any delay could have serious consequences. You should consider how far it is to your nearest hospital and how long it would take to be transferred there in an emergency.
- The risks increase if you have a preexisting medical condition or have experienced complications when giving birth previously, so if your doctor recommends that you give birth in a hospital, it is wise to heed his or her advice.
- Birth is unpredictable, particularly if it's your first time. Try to keep an open mind about your options for pain relief, and remember that if you're having a home birth and decide you do need an epidural, there will be an extra wait while you're transferred to a hospital.

. 56 .
Does walking or squatting speed up labor?

The traditional picture of a laboring woman lying flat on her back, legs in stirrups, screaming in agony, is a far cry from how the majority of women spend the early hours of labor. Increasingly, women are encouraged to stay upright for as long as possible, and even to take a long walk, in the hope that gravity will aid the descent of the baby's head and put pressure on the cervix, encouraging it to open.

So strong is this belief that you may find yourself being marched down the corridor by an eager nurse, even if you'd rather lie down in bed. You may also hear horror stories of how lying down could trigger a downward spiral of medical interventions, starting with you being given drugs to boost the strength of contractions, and ending up with your baby being delivered by forceps or you being wheeled into the operating room for an emergency C-section.

Some studies have found that contractions are stronger when women are upright, compared to when they are lying down, so the thinking goes that labor should progress faster if women are upright. Although this is true to some extent, the effect isn't massive. A review of 21 studies that took in a total of 3,706 women found that, on average, the first stage of labor was an hour shorter in women who were upright, compared to those who lay down (the average first stage of labor is twelve to fourteen hours in first-time moms). Women who remained upright were slightly less likely to request an epidural, but there was no difference in the use of other types of pain relief.

Neither was there much evidence for the idea that lying down would make a natural vaginal birth less likely: Rates of uncomplicated vaginal births and ones involving mechanical help (in the form of forceps or a ventouse) were similar, and although C-sections were slightly less likely among women who remained upright, the difference was small enough that it could have arisen by chance.

Further analysis found that walking wasn't any better than sitting or kneeling upright in bed; it was lying down that made the difference. The authors concluded that women should be encouraged to take up whatever position they find most comfortable during labor, while avoiding spending long periods lying down.

Once you enter the second stage of labor and the baby's head has entered the birth canal, then squatting may slightly speed things along—although whether your leg muscles are strong enough to maintain this position for a long time is another matter. A review of twenty studies found that, on average, the second stage of labor (which usually lasts one to two hours) was reduced by about four and a half minutes in women who assumed an upright or squatting position, compared to those who lay down—although the quality of many of those studies was described as poor. There were fewer episiotomies in women who remained upright, though this was offset by an increase in tears to the tissue between the vagina and back passage.

. 57 .
Should I push?

Another common misconception about labor is that it's all about pushing—particularly as the latest evidence suggests that pushing should be reserved for the final minutes of labor, once the baby's head is already in sight.

Many doctors and midwives believe that pushing as soon as the cervix opens wide enough to let the baby's head through will make birth happen more quickly, especially if a woman has had an epidural and may be less aware of any natural urge to push. That view is being challenged by recent evidence that suggests it may be better to relax and give the baby time to move gently down the birth canal, with women being asked to push only once the head is visible.

Trying to get to the bottom of this issue, an American group recently reviewed seven clinical trials that compared immediate versus delayed pushing in women who had already had an epidural. It found that waiting for up to two hours for the baby to descend before asking women to push decreased the amount of time the women spent pushing and actually increased their chances of having a natural delivery. UK midwives were recently advised to give women with an epidural in place an extra hour to let the baby's head descend, which is an indication that people are starting to take this evidence on board.

Although it has been less well studied, the same principle may also apply to women who haven't had an epidural. A recent trial found that delaying pushing for up to ninety minutes after the cervix had fully dilated roughly halved the total amount of time women spent pushing, without significantly increasing the overall time spent in labor. In other words, you can get there just as quickly with much less effort.

. 58 .
Is it better to tear or be cut in terms of healing?

An Irish stand-up comedian named Dara O'Briain does a sketch about the antenatal classes he and his wife attended when they were expecting their first child. In it, he describes their teacher's account of how, at some point, a choice may need to be made between a cut and a tear. "Obviously," the teacher told them, "you should choose the natural path. Besides which, a tear heals better than a cut." When O'Briain recounted this experience to a friend a few days later, the friend said, "Oh, well, of course, that's well known. Most surgeons these days for the initial incision will use a tear."

I was also told that it would be better to tear, so I was horrified when, after an hour and a half of trying to push my baby out, my midwife turned to me and said, "I think we may have to make a little cut." My reaction was to take a deep breath and push with all my might. Out shot my daughter, and I was left with a second-degree tear that subsequently became infected and took a long time to heal, so the issue of whether it's better to be cut or to tear is one that haunts me to this day.

The answer is nowhere near as clear-cut as you might imagine. During the 1970s, episiotomies (a deliberate cut made in the muscular tissue between the vagina and back passage called the perineum) were performed as a matter of routine in order to protect the anal sphincter muscles that control the bowels and to speed up birth. The problem was that it led to many women being cut unnecessarily and suffering discomfort while the wound healed. Also, episiotomies don't always work, because some women who are cut also tear.

These days, the trend is to let nature take its course and cut a woman only if it seems almost certain that she is going to tear, if the baby is in distress, or if forceps are going to be used. "I can honestly say that I have never met a midwife or obstetrician who claims to have done episiotomies when they thought they were unnecessary," says Philip Steer. "Unfortunately, there is no straightforward way of determining who is going to suffer an anal-sphincter injury other than clinical judgment as to how big the baby is and how tight the perineum is."

The benefit of an episiotomy is that—particularly if the cut is made at an angle rather than straight down the center of the perineum—it can direct the injury away from the anal muscles.

In terms of healing, O'Briain's antenatal teacher wasn't completely off the mark; as a general rule, tissue does heal better when it is torn. During a C-section, many surgeons will use a scalpel to cut through the skin and tough connective tissues and to make a small incision in the muscular wall of the uterus; this is then extended by tearing the tissue. "This separates the tissues along their natural lines and enables them to come together more easily when the wound is closed," says Steer.

The problem with tears in the perineal tissue is that the "natural line" of the tissue often runs straight down the back of the vagina, and—if the tear extends too far—into the back passage. Healing may be less uncomfortable than if an angled cut is made, since there is less tension on the wound when you sit down, but there may be an increased risk of serious injury in a minority of cases. Virginia Beckett, a consultant obstetrician and gynecologist at Bradford Teaching Hospital in the UK and a spokesperson for the Royal College of Obstetricians and Gynaecologists, says, "Personally, I would rather have a nice clean surgical cut that is designed to take pressure away from the important structures down there, than risk an uncontrolled tear, but we don't always get it right."

. 59 .
Does perineal massage work?

In the hope of preventing a tear, I hovered over the bath each morning during the final weeks of pregnancy, diligently rubbing olive oil into the back wall of my vagina. Since no one had coached me on what I should be doing, I simply did what seemed to make the most sense: I focused on relaxing my pelvic-floor muscles and stretching the tissue in the way I assumed it would be stretched when my daughter finally put in an appearance. Perineal massage is neither dignified nor relaxing. So is it worth the effort?

The Cochrane Collaboration recently reviewed four studies in which women who massaged their perineum once or twice a week from thirty-five weeks of pregnancy were compared to those who did nothing. Although perineal massage made no difference in the number of tears, fewer of the women who practiced it required stitches—at least among those women giving birth for the first time. It wasn't a massive difference: Fifteen women would need to massage themselves regularly in order to prevent one woman from being stitched up, but it's better than nothing. Women were also slightly less likely to require an episiotomy. Massaging once or twice a week seemed to be enough, as massaging more frequently didn't improve things.

Unfortunately, perineal massage did nothing to reduce a woman's chances of needing an instrumental delivery (such as one involving forceps or a ventouse) or of developing incontinence; nor did it have any effect on her sexual satisfaction after birth.

If you decide to try perineal massage, here's how to do it:

- Find a comfortable position, such as lying in bed with your legs bent outward, standing with one foot on the edge of the bath or sitting on the toilet.
- Using an unscented natural oil such as olive, sunflower, or sweet almond oil, insert one or both thumbs into the entrance of the vagina.
- Now, pressing down on the back wall, move your thumbs back and forth in a U-shape, focusing on relaxing your muscles at the same time.
- Aim to massage for around five minutes each time. You can try pushing harder each time you do it.

. 60 .
Is there anything else I can do to prevent tearing?

The sad fact is that around 85 percent of women will experience some degree of tearing during a vaginal birth. This can range from minor damage to the skin around the vagina and labia that heals within a couple of days, to the horror of a fourth-degree tear that rips through all the muscles between the vagina and back passage. Fortunately, fourth-degree tears are relatively rare, affecting just 3 to 4 percent of women. But tearing is particularly common in first-time moms, if you have a large baby or one in a difficult position, or if forceps are used to get the baby out.

Is there any way of preventing or minimizing the damage you might suffer? The Cochrane Collaboration recently reviewed different techniques that midwives sometimes use to reduce the risk of tearing, including massaging the perineum (see 59: "Does perineal massage work?"), applying a warm compress, placing pressure on the perineum, or manipulating the baby's head to slow the rate at which it emerges.

What seemed to be most effective was applying a warm compress to the perineum during the second stage of labor, when women are actively pushing. This reduced the risk of serious tearing, helped to relieve pain, and reduced the risk of urinary incontinence. Giving birth in water also seems to reduce the chances that a woman will need an episiotomy, though the risk of a serious tear remains about the same.

Although the idea of tearing during childbirth may make you cringe, recovering from a tear isn't as bad as you might imagine (see 70: "How do I know if my stitches are okay?").

. 61 .
Will delaying cord-clamping benefit my baby?

A proud new father is handed a pair of scissors and asked if he'd like to cut the umbilical cord. Should he do it or allow the lifeline that has connected mother and baby for the past nine months to pulsate for just a few minutes more?

Once the baby is safely delivered and starts breathing air, the umbilical cord fast becomes redundant. A series of contractions quickly shuts off the flow of blood to the placenta, which then begins to detach from the uterus wall and follows the baby out into the big, wide world.

In many Western countries, midwives are quick to clamp and cut the umbilical cord. But the placenta contains a large amount of the baby's blood, and some have argued that this blood should be given two to three minutes to flow back into the baby's body before the cord is cut. Doing so can increase a newborn's blood volume by around 32 percent.

Others argue that this extra blood isn't necessarily good for babies: They take longer than adults to dispose of worn-out red blood cells, which can lead to a buildup of a yellow pigment called bilirubin that becomes toxic at high levels and leads to jaundice. However, iron deficiency is common among babies during the first few months of life, and any extra blood they receive at birth should help counter it. Around 9 percent of young children in the U.S. are thought to be deficient in iron, and that can have a negative impact on brain development.

Several recent studies have bolstered support for waiting a few minutes before clamping and cutting the cord. In one of the largest studies to date, Swedish experts compared four hundred babies whose cords were clamped either ten seconds or three minutes after birth. Four months later, the babies whose cords had been clamped later had higher iron levels and were less likely to be suffering from iron deficiency or anemia. There was no difference in rates of jaundice between the two groups.

A separate review of eleven studies by the Cochrane Collaboration found higher levels of iron in babies whose cords were clamped later, but this time there was an increase in the number of those who needed treatment for jaundice (which usually involves placing a baby under a blanket that bathes the skin in light and helps break down the bilirubin). The authors concluded that so long as access to jaundice treatment is readily available, then delayed cord-clamping should be offered more widely.

Ouch!

What's more painful: childbirth or having your leg chopped off?

Just how painful is labor? It's a question most women ponder at some point during pregnancy. If you're deliberately trying not to think about it, then I advise you to skip this section.

Personally, I can say that nothing I've experienced compares with the pain of labor, in both intensity and type of pain. It's not like the throb of a headache, the shooting pain of standing on a badly sprained ankle, or the raw, searing pain of a bad burn. The experience also seems to vary from woman to woman. Although almost all women will experience lower abdominal pain during contractions, some may also experience continuous lower-back pain or pain in other highly focused areas. The pain occurs for lots of reasons: intense muscle contractions, the stretching and tearing of internal tissues, and pressure on the joints of the pelvis.

There's a tendency for antenatal teachers to gloss over the intensity of labor pain, which I think is a mistake, as at least one study has suggested that women whose expectations of labor are violated by the reality of it feel more pain. A recent study of 324 pregnant women found that though 36 percent anticipated suffering extreme pain during labor, 65 percent reported experiencing it. If women aren't given accurate information about what they can expect from labor, it is impossible for them to make an informed decision about preferences for pain relief. On the other hand, fear about pain can make it worse, and I certainly don't mean to scare people. The reality is that labor hurts, but it's not insurmountable, and there are coping strategies and drugs that can help you through (see 65: "Can hypnosis or alternative therapies reduce labor pain?").

Can men ever hope to understand the pain of childbirth? The answer is: maybe. Back in 1981, a pain researcher named Ronald Melzack and his colleagues at McGill University in Canada set out to assess labor pain in 141 women and compare it to other types of pain such as back pain, nonterminal cancer pain, or toothache. They used something called the McGill Pain Questionnaire, a list of seventy-eight adjectives divided into twenty groups that describe different aspects of pain. Patients are asked to circle adjectives to describe how they are feeling: words like "jumping," "flashing," "shooting," "cutting," or "lacerating." Each of the words has been given a numerical score; when they are added together, the result provides a good idea of how much pain someone is in.

Melzack gave the questionnaire to women whose contractions were under five minutes apart and whose cervixes had dilated two to three centimeters. Over 33 percent of the women used the following words to describe their pain: "sharp," "cramping," "aching," "throbbing," "stabbing," "hot," "shooting," and "heavy." "Intense" and "tight" were widely used, and over 80 percent of women said their pain was either "tiring" or "exhausting."

A later study by the same group found that 60 percent of first-time moms described the pain of contractions as being "unbearable," "intolerable," "extremely severe," or "excruciating."

The researchers found widespread variation in overall pain scores between individuals. Women who suffered from premenstrual pain seemed to have a particularly hard time of it, possibly because their bodies overproduce chemicals called prostaglandins, which help to trigger contractions. In addition, first-time moms seemed to suffer more pain than women who had been through labor before, and pain scores were marginally lower for women who had attended antenatal classes that included information about breathing exercises and relaxation. Other studies have found that first-time moms report more labor pain, particularly during the early stages of labor, when the lower half of the uterus and cervix is being stretched and pulled apart. It's possible that these areas are more supple and transmit fewer pain signals in existing mothers.

So how does the pain of labor compare to other types of pain? When Melzack compared scores from patients battling other conditions or illnesses, labor pain ranked as more painful than nonterminal cancer pain, back pain, toothache, or arthritis. But it could be worse: A different study found that having a limb amputated, or a rare condition called causalgia (in which the arms and legs feel as if they are continuously burning and aching), ranked worse than the pain of labor.

. 63 .
Do hormones block the pain of labor?

Advocates of natural childbirth insist that the body produces natural painkillers during labor, and to some extent they're correct: Contractions do trigger the release of hormones such as beta-endorphin, which binds to and blocks the same receptors in the brain as morphine. The release of beta-endorphin is dampened in women who receive epidural anesthesia primarily because their bodies are no longer screaming out for pain relief.

Israeli researchers recently found that women's pain tolerance increases during labor, which could be because of chemicals such as beta-endorphin. They used a device called a dolorimeter, which applies steady pressure to tender areas of the body and records the point at which it becomes painful, to record pain thresholds in forty pregnant women before, during, and after birth. Women experienced significant increases in their pain threshold once labor was established, and this was especially true of women whose pregnancies had lasted forty weeks or more. Just why women whose pregnancies reached full term should have greater pain tolerance is unclear, though studies in rats have shown increases in pain tolerance in the days leading up to labor as well as during the actual event.

In a separate study, Danish researchers found that women's pain thresholds increased during the third trimester. In addition, the intensity of labor pain was lower in women who had experienced pelvic pain recently—possibly because the body's natural mechanisms for relieving pain were already activated.

Labor triggers the release of the fight-or-flight hormones adrenaline (epinephrine) and noradrenaline. Often perceived as the bad guys because they can reduce the intensity of contractions, these also reduce pain. One evolutionary explanation for why we release these hormones during labor is that by slowing labor, they might buy women some extra time to seek out a safe and sheltered place to give birth.

Just like beta-endorphin, levels of adrenaline and noradrenaline fall once women are given drugs to relieve pain, but that's not necessarily a bad thing, as women often find that labor progresses more quickly once their pain is under control. However, since panic can also increase the release of adrenaline, it is worth trying other coping techniques such as breathing and relaxation.

Finally, other studies have suggested that a lack of family support can heighten women's perception of pain. Women who give birth during the morning seem to experience less pain than those who give birth at night, possibly due to natural variations in the levels of hormones at different times of day. So, if you can manage it, aim to get a good night's rest and plenty of hugs from your partner, and hope for the best.

. 64 .
Why do women come back for more?

How many times have you been told: "Once you hold your baby in your arms you'll forget all about the pain you have just endured"?

Although it's not true to say that labor pain is forgotten immediately, the memory of it does seem to fade with time—at least in women who have a positive experience of childbirth. Women who describe childbirth as a negative experience two months after giving birth tend to have fewer subsequent children and take longer to have their next child than those with positive memories.

In a recent study, Swedish researchers asked women to rate their labor pain on a seven-point scale at two months, one year, and five years after the birth. Those who, at two months, had a very positive or positive recollection of childbirth remembered the pain as less intense as the months went by, suggesting that the memories were edited over time, while women who described childbirth as a negative experience didn't change their assessment of labor pain at later dates. Importantly, whether women rated childbirth as positive or negative was unrelated to the amount of pain they had experienced. Instead, it seemed to come down to other factors, such as the level of support they received from the doctors, nurses, and midwives looking after them.

There's a physical mechanism by which childbirth might muddy our memories of the experience. Oxytocin, which is released in vast quantities during late pregnancy and childbirth, seems to alter the way in which memories are laid down. Although no one has specifically studied the effect of this hormone on memories of childbirth, other studies in which people have inhaled oxytocin before doing memory tests have suggested that it can reduce the ability to recall lists of words or pictures, while animal studies have hinted that oxytocin can interfere with the consolidation and retrieval of memories. If this is true, it might suggest that pregnancy-related forgetfulness, or "momnesia," has an upside: helping women to forget the pain of labor.

. 65 .
Can hypnosis or alternative therapies reduce labor pain?

Despite growing numbers of C-sections in many Western countries, natural childbirth methods such as massage, birthing pools, and hypnosis are increasingly popular. However, because many of these therapies have never been rigorously tested, it can be difficult to know if they are any better than a placebo or nothing at all.

Partly for this reason, the Cochrane Collaboration recently pulled together all its previous studies assessing different methods of pain relief during labor (reviewing 310 studies in all). These methods ranged from established medical procedures such as epidurals to injections of sterile water, hypnosis, and massage.

The methods were divided into three categories: those that work, those that may work, and those about which there is insufficient evidence to make a judgment. Things that definitely provide pain relief include epidurals and gas and air; none of the nondrug methods made the grade. Water births, relaxation, acupuncture, and massage made it into the "what may work" category. In most cases, only a single good-quality clinical trial was available to make the judgment, but these methods do seem to relieve pain and improve the experience of childbirth compared to placebo or nothing at all.

In the case of hypnosis, sterile-water injections, aromatherapy, TENS (transcutaneous electrical nerve stimulation), biofeedback, and opioid drugs like Demerol, the Cochrane Collaboration said there wasn't sufficient evidence to judge effectiveness. That's not to say they don't work, but any studies that exist aren't of good enough quality to prove it.

Let's look at the evidence for some of these alternative methods of pain relief in more detail.

Water birth

Once dismissed as a fad, birth pools are now a common fixture of labor wards in many countries, particularly the UK, where more than three quarters of hospitals now provide them. American hospitals have been slower to embrace the concept of water birth, although a growing number of hospitals and birthing centers provide them. Supporters argue that warm water relieves the pain of contractions, reduces the risk of tearing, and helps women feel more in control of their birth. Fears do remain about women getting too hot or too cold and of babies being at greater risk of infection or drowning if they are born in water. In the majority of cases, women who use birthing pools get out of the water before giving birth, making some of these concerns irrelevant. Of the studies that have been conducted, there is no convincing evidence of any increased risk of complications among women who give birth in water.

When the Cochrane Collaboration reviewed twelve studies looking at the effects of immersion in warm water, it concluded that although it made no difference to the rates of C-section, instrumental delivery (involving forceps or a ventouse), the baby's health, or the risk of tearing, it did reduce the intensity of pain, and women were more likely to feel satisfied with their birth experience.

Transcutaneous Electrical Nerve Stimulation (TENS)

TENS machines comprise a small box that transmits low-intensity electrical impulses to the skin via several electrodes, which are usually attached to the lower back, producing a kind of buzzing sensation. Although TENS is very popular in the UK, with most pharmacies offering machines for hire, TENS is less well known in the U.S. No one really understands why TENS works, but one theory is that the electrical pulses stimulate nerves in the spinal cord that block the transmission of pain. It may also serve as a distraction and give women a sense of control over their contractions.

Though plenty of clinical trials have investigated whether TENS works for labor pain, and a handful of these studies have found some benefit, the majority have found none. For this reason, the UK's National Institute for Health and Clinical Excellence, which issues evidence-based guidelines for doctors, recently stated that TENS shouldn't be recommended for pain relief in labor. The Cochrane Collaboration, which looked at seventeen of these studies, also concluded that TENS had little or no effect on pain intensity or on women's satisfaction with pain relief.

Massage

If you attend antenatal classes, you'll probably be shown some massage techniques that can be helpful during labor. A common one is for the birth partner to use the heel of the hand or the thumbs to firmly massage around the base of the spine, which supposedly counters the pain of contractions. A shoulder or back massage may also help to relax you during labor. When the Cochrane team reviewed six trials looking at whether massage relieves labor pain, they found some reduction in pain during the first stage of labor, but no effect later on.

Acupuncture and acupressure

Acupuncture points commonly used to reduce labor pain are located on the hands, feet, and ears—although a scientific explanation for how acupuncture works is still lacking.

The Cochrane Review examined thirteen studies and found that both acupuncture and acupressure reduced the intensity of pain and increased women's satisfaction with pain relief. They were also associated with fewer instrumental deliveries (involving forceps or a ventouse) and fewer C-sections. Though that may sound impressive, just three of the thirteen trials looked at the risk of instrumental deliveries, and just one trial of 120 women recorded the rate of C-sections. Differences between the studies that looked at pain relief also made it difficult to say with any certainty just how effective acupuncture is. Other reviews have similarly concluded that more research is needed.

Hypnosis

Hypno-birthing is a form of self-hypnosis in which you are trained to relax and visualize yourself in another place, such as a beautiful garden, or picture a dial that you can turn up or down to reduce sensation in your body. Women are taught breathing techniques to calm themselves and aid pushing, and they're encouraged to substitute words such as "pressure" for "pain," and "surges" for "contractions." The main goal is to reduce tension and fear in the hope that birth will progress more naturally; despite being "hypnotized," women remain fully in control and aware of what is going on around them.

Having used hypno-birthing myself, I can testify that it reduced my anxiety in the run-up to labor, though I'm not sure it was helpful during labor itself. When things got really bad, I was impelled to throw a sponge at the MP3 player that told me for the hundredth time to "embrace each gentle birthing wave."

The few studies that have investigated hypnosis during childbirth tend to agree. Although one Cochrane review of five studies found a decreased use of pain-relief drugs and a greater likelihood of a natural vaginal birth among women who used hypnosis, when the Cochrane Collaboration conducted its review of reviews, it found no difference in women's satisfaction with pain relief or the childbirth experience compared to women who weren't hypnotized.

Relaxation and yoga

Relaxation techniques such as progressive muscle relaxation and yoga do seem to show some benefit, similar to hypnosis. A review of eleven studies of relaxation techniques found that they reduced the intensity of pain and increased women's satisfaction with their pain relief, as well as improving their satisfaction with birth overall.

Aromatherapy

The Cochrane Collaboration found just two good-quality studies looking at the effectiveness of aromatherapy for pain management during labor. These studies, which compared aromatherapy to placebo or no treatment, found no difference in the intensity of pain or the likelihood of having a vaginal birth or a C-section. Nor was there any difference in the use of additional drugs by women in the different groups.

. 66 .
Does an epidural make a C-section more likely?

Most doctors and midwives agree that, by far, the most effective means of reducing pain in labor is epidural anesthesia. Those who have succumbed to the lumbar needle will testify to the enormous wave of relief that comes with the elimination of hours of exhausting pain. Yet lingering doubts about the safety of epidurals for mothers and babies remain. Some mothers worry that it may increase their risk of a C-section or delivery involving forceps or make it more likely that they will tear. Others worry about the drugs reaching the baby and harming it in some way.

Some women feel that requesting an epidural would be a kind of failure, because it means they couldn't handle the pain. One friend told me that she didn't think she'd be able to look her antenatal classmates in the eye if she had an epidural, never mind the fact that, statistically, many of them were likely to do exactly the same thing. Around 58 percent of U.S. women have an epidural, while in the UK, it is closer to 20 percent.

Labor is one of the most painful experiences that you're ever likely to go through (see 62: "What's more painful: childbirth or having your leg chopped off?"). It varies a great deal from woman to woman and from pregnancy to pregnancy. Some women undoubtedly give birth without tremendous pain, but others need drugs to get through it. If you've never been through labor, it is impossible to know how your body will react, so it is best to keep an open mind about the options available to you.

A recent study of women who made birth plans in advance of labor found that although over half of them originally said they'd like to avoid having an epidural, 65 percent ultimately requested one. What's more, 90 percent of women who received an epidural reported being pleased with their decision when asked about it later.

An epidural is an injection administered via a tube inserted into the lower spine, close to the nerves that transmit pain signals from the lower body up to the brain. This may sound gruesome, but it isn't as painful as you might imagine (particularly when you're already in the throes of labor), and you're usually given a small injection of local anesthetic before the tube goes in. Drugs that inhibit those pain signals are then pumped into the spine, providing rapid relief from labor pain. Because the drugs are injected locally, they don't get into the baby's body.

Whereas having an epidural used to mean that you'd be flat on the bed and unable to move your lower body for the rest of labor, modern drug combinations mean that, though you're unlikely to be running around the labor ward, you can get into different birthing positions, such as on hands and knees, and to bear down and push your baby out during the second stage of labor. Women are often given a handheld pump with which they can increase levels of the anesthetic drugs and control the amount of sensation they feel.

There are some risks, such as the epidural not working properly, a sudden drop in blood pressure, or the accidental puncture of the tough envelope surrounding the spinal cord, which can trigger headaches. Women may lose the ability to sense when their bladder is full, so a catheter is usually inserted (also not as bad as it sounds).

Like so many areas of pregnancy and birth, those studies that have compared the risks of epidural anesthesia with births without any drugs have reached mixed conclusions, depending on the type of women they studied and the precise question asked. The Cochrane Collaboration recently brought together the results of twenty-three of these studies to try to reach some kind of consensus on the risks and benefits of epidurals. It concluded that they do not increase the risk of C-section, the length of the first stage of labor, long-term backache, or have any negative effects on the baby. However, the second stage of labor may last slightly longer (around thirteen minutes, on average); women are marginally more likely to need supplemental oxytocin to boost the strength of contractions; and they are 42 percent more likely to have an instrumental delivery (one involving forceps or a ventouse).

Because the chances of having an instrumental delivery are pretty low (only around 4 percent of births involve forceps and 8 percent a ventouse), this isn't as bad as it sounds. I contacted the authors of the review and asked them to calculate how many women would need to be given an epidural before one of them had an instrumental delivery as a result. The answer is approximately twenty.

Even so, you may feel nervous about any increased risk, because instrumental deliveries tend to be associated with a greater chance of tearing or a cut being required in the wall of the vagina in order to help the baby out. But even though slightly more women who have epidurals have an instrumental delivery, that doesn't necessarily mean the epidural is to blame. Women who already have an epidural in place are more likely to be offered mechanical help to get the baby out because their vaginal area is already numb.

A separate study that examined the main risk factors for serious injuries to the anal-sphincter muscle that controls the bowels found no association with either epidural anesthesia or the use of oxytocin to speed up or induce labor.

As for risks to the baby, the Cochrane review found that newborns whose mothers had epidurals in place showed fewer signs of distress (as measured by a fall in blood pH called acidosis), although there was no difference in more severe cases. Nor was there any difference in admissions to the intensive care unit between the babies of mothers who had epidurals or no pain relief, or in their Apgar score (a measure of how healthy the baby looks when it is first delivered).

. 67 .
Do gas and air or Demerol relieve pain?

Besides epidurals, the most common drugs offered to women in labor are gas and air (nitrous oxide) and Demerol. Nitrous oxide works not by interfering with the transmission of pain signals to the brain but by making you less bothered by them. It is the most commonly used drug for relieving labor pain and helps take the edge off contractions, but it can leave you feeling light-headed and sick if you inhale too much of it. The good news is that the effects of the drug wear off quickly, and it doesn't affect the baby. A recent review concluded that fewer women who inhaled nitrous oxide reported experiencing severe or extreme pain during the first stage of labor, compared to those inhaling a placebo drug, which suggests that it does work.

The evidence that Demerol provides effective relief from labor pain is more mixed. Demerol has been available to midwives since the 1950s and is related to the powerful painkiller morphine—though it is certainly less effective than that. It is injected into the muscles; unlike nitrous oxide or an epidural, it can cross the placenta and make babies sleepier, less good at suckling, and slower to establish breast-feeding. Large doses can interfere with the baby's breathing and muscle movement, although it is generally regarded as safe for use in labor, and drugs can be given to reverse its effects in the unlikely event of an overdose. Demerol tends to make you feel drowsy and can make you feel sick or dizzy.

When the same review looked at studies of Demerol, it concluded that there was insufficient evidence to judge whether it was more effective than a placebo or other interventions for pain relief in labor. This may seem incredible for a drug that has been around for so long and is used in 39 to 56 percent of obstetric units in the U.S., but few high-quality studies have ever been done to establish if it really works. Those that have been conducted have produced mixed results, with some saying it has no effect and others suggesting that it does have a modest effect.

The Post-Pregnancy Body

. 68 .
What causes the baby blues?

It's ironic that, at what could be one of the happiest and most exciting times of a woman's life, she can be sent plummeting into the depths of despair. Yet up to 13 percent of new mothers experience postnatal depression, and 70 percent experience the more short-lived symptoms of the baby blues, including extreme sadness, mood swings, anxiety, sleeplessness, and irritability. I remember being overwhelmed with a sense of not being able to cope and feeling an irrational anger at my husband when he left the house for a couple of hours a week after the birth of our daughter (even though she was sound asleep). Several friends who had babies at the same time later admitted to feelings of depression in the immediate aftermath of birth—despite putting a brave face on it at the time. Fortunately for all of us, it was a passing phase, but it was only as we prepared for our next round of births that we felt comfortable enough to talk openly about what we went through the first time around.

Only about a quarter of women seek professional help for depressive symptoms after birth. Yet not taking these feelings seriously can have disastrous consequences in terms of women's ability to bond with their child and their own long-term mental health. Children of depressed mothers tend to be more withdrawn, and women who have suffered from postnatal depression are twice as likely to experience another depressive episode within the next five years.

What's to blame for this often extreme crash in mood? Unsurprisingly, hormones play a big part. In the first three to four days after birth, levels of estrogen drop a hundred- to a thousand-fold, and there are also big falls in progesterone.

Julia Sacher and her colleagues at the Max Planck Institute in Leipzig, Germany, recently discovered that this fall in estrogen corresponds with a dramatic rise in levels of an enzyme called monoamine oxidase A (MAO-A) in the brain, which breaks down several mood-boosting chemicals, including serotonin, dopamine, and noradrenaline. Sacher found that levels of MAO-A peaked five days after birth, which is precisely when many women experience the greatest crash in mood. Although it was a small study, those women with the greatest rise in MAO-A seemed to be at the greatest risk of going on to develop postnatal depression. Other studies have found that women who experience severe symptoms of baby blues in the first week after birth are at a higher risk of developing longer-term depression. Sacher suggests that eating foods that are rich in the amino acids tryptophan and tyrosine (such as wheat, oats, red meat, and seafood) may help reduce the risk, as both are needed to make mood-boosting chemicals such as serotonin. However, if a woman continues to feel depressed or unable to cope much beyond ten days after the birth (when symptoms of the baby blues typically lift), she should speak to a doctor.

. 69 .
Why can't I poop?

Constipation is a common side effect of giving birth that few women are warned about. It could be two to three days before you have a BM, and especially if you've experienced a tear, have become dehydrated as a result of a long labor or losing blood, or didn't eat much fiber in the run-up to birth, that first trip to the bathroom can become a mental battleground. Even if you aren't constipated, it may take a while to poop, because pregnancy hormones such as progesterone and the birth itself slow down the movement of digested food through the gut. In addition, the bowels can open during a natural birth (whether or not you are aware of it), which adds to the delay of needing to go.

I had terrible constipation following my first birth, and too embarrassed to say anything to the midwives who came to visit me, I suffered in silence. The result was an anal fissure: a painful tear in the wall of my bottom, which, in combination with the vaginal tear I'd experienced giving birth, led to long-term problems that ultimately required surgery to correct. I write this not to scare people but in the hope that others can avoid similar misfortune. If you can't go, you're not alone.

One study of 313 women giving birth for the first time found that twenty-nine (9 percent) developed an anal fissure, although few of these would have been diagnosed under normal circumstances, as the symptoms are similar to hemorrhoids, and most eventually clear up by themselves (I was particularly unlucky). Less serious consequences of not pooping include abdominal pain and increased discomfort when you do go.

You can avoid constipation by drinking plenty of fluids and eating lots of fresh fruit and vegetables. Once constipation develops, you need to try to go to the toilet as soon as the urge takes you, even if the prospect is terrifying. "Women are often fearful of opening their bowels after birth because they think it will be painful, so they withhold it, and it gets more difficult as a result," says Virginia Beckett. "It becomes a self-fulfilling prophecy."

Besides staying hydrated, Beckett suggests taking a stool softener such as lactulose (you can ask your doctor for a prescription) if you haven't opened your bowels twenty-four to forty-eight hours after the birth.

If you're struggling to go, experts recommend sitting on the toilet, ideally with your feet on a footstool and your elbows resting on your knees, and relaxing. If nothing happens, you can try to stimulate bowel movements by doing an exercise called bracing and bulging. Put one hand on your lower abdomen and one on your waist, and then tighten your abdominal muscles: You should feel your hands being pushed out forwards and sideways (this is a brace). Now do the opposite and push your tummy muscles out to the front (this is a bulge). Repeat ten times, ending with a big bulge. If you're still getting nowhere, don't be embarrassed to speak to a doctor or midwife about your problem.

. 70 .
How do I know if my stitches are okay?

Around a third of women who have a vaginal birth will experience a tear that needs to be stitched up afterward—another fact frequently shrouded in silence. Though the prospect of needing stitches in such an intimate area may sound terrifying to the uninitiated, the reality is that, although uncomfortable, the pain of stitches isn't unbearable, and in the vast majority of cases, women heal just fine.

A second-degree tear (one involving the skin and muscle behind the vagina but not extending into the muscles around the back passage) will typically take two to three weeks to heal, but the initial pain should have eased after several days. "A week to ten days after the birth, you should be feeling markedly better," says Beckett. Beckett warns that you may feel a slight "tightening" sensation around the wound shortly before the stitches dissolve at around ten days as the tissues knit together and start to heal, but this is normal. However, if you start to feel unwell, experience significantly increased pain or heat around the wound, or notice a smelly discharge, you should speak to a doctor or midwife, as you may have developed an infection. The risk of developing one can be reduced by keeping the wound as clean and dry as possible (which is admittedly difficult, given the location); an infection can be treated using antibiotics. Beckett recommends sitting in a shallow bath of warm water two to three times a day (you don't need to add anything to the water) and patting the area dry afterward.

Given how common stitches are, little research has been done on the most effective way of relieving the inevitable discomfort. Women are told to use ice packs or cool gel pads to reduce pain and swelling, but a recent Cochrane review concluded that the degree of pain relief was small. Meanwhile, different doctors and midwives may recommend applying witch hazel or adding salt, lavender oil, or arnica to the bath, though there's little evidence to suggest that any one of these methods is better than another. Acetaminophen or ibuprofen can be taken to relieve the pain, and both are considered safe for the baby, as is diclofenac (although this has to be prescribed by a doctor). Doing pelvic-floor exercises and avoiding sitting for long periods can improve circulation to the area and may speed up healing. Probably the best thing is to try a combination of strategies and see what works for you.

Although the initial pain of a tear should have subsided after a week, it is quite normal to feel some discomfort in the area surrounding the vagina for weeks or even months after a natural birth. If this is distressing you or affecting your sex life, you should speak to a doctor (see 54: "Are vaginal births really better than C-sections?").

Even if you don't need stitches, it's usual for the whole vaginal area to feel swollen and tender for a few days after a vaginal birth.

. 71 .
Can other countries (for example, France) teach us anything about getting back into shape after birth?

We often envy the French: They generally have better food and are more chic. But there's one area where we genuinely should feel green-eyed: postnatal care.

In many countries, women are discharged from the hospital and left largely to themselves. In France, women see a gynecologist within the first month of birth, when they're able to discuss any pain or sexual problems they're experiencing. They also routinely get twelve half-hour sessions with a postnatal physiotherapist who specializes in rehabilitating the pelvic-floor and abdominal muscles.

"We focus on bringing the perineum back to health and improving sexual sensation," says James Turgis, a French physiotherapist who now runs a private physiotherapy clinic called Mummy's Physio in London. The abdominal muscles will be checked for any damage or separation, and women are given exercises to tone them up. It's no wonder French women are back in their pre-pregnancy jeans before they know it (mine are languishing sadly at the back of the wardrobe).

Although it's normal for the skin of your belly to feel a bit saggy in the months after birth, some women develop "mommy tummy," a horizontal roll of fat that hangs down in two horns if you bend over. This is a sign that the abdominal muscles have failed to close back together after pregnancy (the technical name is an abdominal diastasis). As the baby grows during pregnancy, the muscle that wraps around the front of the belly begins to pull apart. In a few countries, including France and Australia, the extent of the damage is checked before women leave the hospital, and they are given exercises to correct it. In other countries, this simple test is overlooked, and women go home oblivious.

Besides causing mommy tummy, an untreated diastasis can lead to lower-back pain and bladder incontinence, and if women start to exercise with a diastasis, it can cause further problems. "Unless the tummy muscles have closed back together, then the pelvic-floor muscles don't have a good anchor," says Maria Elliott, a physiotherapist who runs SimplyWomensHealth on London's Harley Street. "Many women who were fit before birth consider their stomach muscles are really strong and mistakenly go out running or start exercising and develop problems like stress incontinence."

Doing sit-ups or abdominal crunches before the tummy gap has closed can cause the muscles to pull even farther apart. "In France, women are initially helped to strengthen pelvic-floor muscles and to close the tummy gap. Once this is achieved, they are able to start abdominal exercises," says Elliott.

The good news is that you can check your abdominal muscles yourself. To do this, lie flat on your back with your knees bent, put your fingers into your belly button or just above it, and press down as you start to roll your head and shoulders up off the floor. You should feel the two sides of the muscle pressing together, and you should be able to get only the tip of one or two fingers into that gap. If the gap is much bigger, you should consult a doctor or physiotherapist. Problems are more common if you've had more than one baby or if your baby was particularly big. If you do discover a gap between your muscles, there are some simple exercises to help close it:

- Lie on your back with your knees bent, and using your hands or a scarf wrapped around your waist, push your abdominal muscles together. Now, keeping your shoulders pressed into the floor, lift your head, exhaling as you do so. Return your head to the floor. Do fifty reps twice a day.
- Still on your back, tilt your pelvis up toward your head and pull your abdominal muscles in while keeping your buttocks relaxed. Then roll your pelvis back down and relax. Repeat ten to fifteen times.
- In the same position, with your abdominals pulled in, add a load by sliding one heel down until your leg is flat on the floor, then slide it back up again. Now do the same on the other side. Repeat ten to fifteen times with each leg.
- Move onto your hands and knees and relax your stomach muscles. As you exhale, pull your belly button up into your body as tight as it can go, drawing your pelvic-floor muscles in at the same time. Hold for about ten seconds, breathing normally, then relax and repeat one more time.

Pregnancy also takes its toll on the pelvic-floor muscles. "The hormonal changes during the first three months of pregnancy can change the pelvic-floor muscles, never mind whether there has been a C-section or a vaginal delivery," says Stephanie Prendergast, a physiotherapist at the Pelvic Health and Rehabilitation Center in San Francisco. The muscles may be overstretched and sluggish, or too tight. Conventional pelvic-floor exercises will lift and strengthen the muscles (see 26: "How do I know if I'm doing my pelvic-floor exercises properly?"), but women with very tight muscles also need to stretch and lengthen them, or such exercises won't have the desired effect.

Massaging the whole area from the bikini line right down and around to where the leg meets the buttocks can help improve blood flow and relax muscles. Elliott says that with the right attention and exercise, most women can return to normal and enjoy a healthy sex life again.

. 72 .
Is it normal to be turned off by sex after birth?

Up to 86 percent of women report sexual problems in the first few months after giving birth, and this is more likely if you have experienced a bad tear. Things should improve with time, but when 481 British women were interviewed six months after birth, 64 percent said they were still experiencing at least one sexual problem. Vaginal dryness, pain, and loss of desire were the most common problems, and most women reported having less sex than before having children, especially less oral sex.

Besides damage to the vagina, breast-feeding can wreak havoc. Many women feel like the breasts are sexual "no-go" areas during nursing, while the hormone changes that allow you to breast-feed in the first place can cause the vagina to feel dry and sex to be uncomfortable. The breast-feeding hormone prolactin decreases sex drive, while testosterone, which usually boosts sex drive, is suppressed in both men and women after birth.

That's before you consider the extreme tiredness that comes with feeding through the night and the massive emotional changes that come with giving birth and getting used to your post-pregnancy body. In other words, it's perfectly natural not to feel like having sex.

Remember though, that the hormone changes and the sleep deprivation are temporary. Research suggests that many women don't fully regain their sex drive until their baby reaches one, and feeling guilty about not having sex only makes things worse. It's important to keep talking to each other, and even when your baby is older you may need to be creative about making time for sex.

. 73 .
Is there anything I can do to keep my breasts from sagging after breast-feeding?

Sagging breasts are a battle scar of childbearing that most women see as inevitable. Around three quarters of moms believe their breasts are different after pregnancy, with bigger breasts, loss of firmness, and shrinking breasts being the most frequent complaints.

Most blame breast-feeding for these changes. The UK website Mumsnet has at least four threads devoted to the question "Does breast-feeding make your boobs sag or shrink?" Together they have generated more than 347 responses, mostly from women complaining about the effect that breast-feeding has had on their bodies. "Women consulting a plastic surgeon will often attribute the loss of breast shape or volume to breast-feeding, and concerns over changes in breast appearance are consistently ranked among the most important reasons women elect not to breast-feed their infants," says Brian Rinker, professor of plastic surgery at the University of Kentucky in Lexington.

Surprisingly, breast-feeding isn't the true culprit. At least two studies of women describing breast changes after pregnancy have found that breast-feeding wasn't a significant factor, as women who didn't breast-feed also described their breasts as different. "We found that pregnancy was strongly associated with sagging, and this effect got worse with more pregnancies," says Rinker, who led one of the studies. "Being heavier, having larger breasts, and cigarette smoking were also associated with more sagging, but a history of breast-feeding, curiously, was not."

So how does pregnancy cause the breasts to sag? Regardless of whether you breast-feed, the breasts go through big structural changes during pregnancy that can stretch the skin and ligaments. As early as six to eight weeks, you may notice your cup size beginning to increase; as pregnancy progresses, the network of lobes and ducts that eventually produce milk begins to grow and mature. By the end of the second trimester, the breasts are already up to the task of producing milk, but high levels of the hormone progesterone inhibit it. Progesterone falls once the baby is born, and levels of the breast-feeding hormone prolactin increase, ramping up milk production.

When women stop breast-feeding, these physical changes begin to reverse themselves through a process called involution. First, milk-producing cells begin to self-combust; then the connective tissue surrounding these cells gets remodeled and replaced with fat. This remodeling continues as women age and progress through menopause, when some notice that their breasts shrink in size.

Just how quickly this all happens varies from woman to woman. Some find that their breasts end up smaller after pregnancy. Precisely why this happens to some women and not others is unclear, but experts suspect it may come down to how easily you lay down fat on your breasts, which may compensate for lost breast tissue.

Although it's possible that wearing a supportive bra during pregnancy may help guard against future breast sag or tissue loss, Rinker is skeptical: "I think the major factors are genetics, age, and pregnancy. I don't think exercise or consistent bra use can really help."

. 74 .
Do women who breast-feed really lose their baby weight faster than those who bottle-feed?

Most women gain around nine pounds of fat during pregnancy—usually on their hips and thighs—which is thought to serve as an energy store for breast-feeding once the baby is born. Breast-feeding is frequently touted as a means of shedding this baby weight once pregnancy is over, as exclusive breast-feeding eats up around 595 calories per day during the first two months, and 670 calories after that.

The trouble is, we're told to eat extra calories to make sure our milk supplies don't dry up, never mind that breast-feeding can make you ravenously hungry (and it's not just greed; the breast-feeding hormone prolactin boosts appetite).

So does breast-feeding really help you shed those excess pounds? Although a number of studies have looked into this issue, the conclusions have been less certain than the pro-breast-feeding lobby might have us believe. One problem is that many studies have used moms' own estimates of their weight before and after pregnancy, rather than measuring it directly. Even in studies that have found a link between exclusive breast-feeding and weight loss, the effect is pretty small. A review of five studies that directly weighed and measured women at various points after birth found that after twelve months, the difference in weight loss between women who breast-fed the longest and those who didn't breast-feed at all ranged from 1.3 pounds to 4.4 pounds.

If you do decide to breast-feed and want to speed up your weight loss, the good news is that it can be done without compromising your milk supply. One study found that limiting calorie intake to around 2,092 calories a day (which is roughly what a healthy woman should have been eating before pregnancy if she wasn't dieting), combined with around forty-five minutes of aerobic exercise four times a week, should enable women to lose roughly one pound per week without affecting milk supply, although it would be sensible to wait for your body to recover and for breast-feeding to become properly established before attempting to do it.

. 75 .
Do cells from my baby live on in my body after birth?

Having a baby changes you in more ways than you might imagine. From early pregnancy, you will forever carry a little piece of your baby around with you in the form of fetal cells that continue to circulate in your blood and survive in your bone marrow. Precisely what these cells are doing remains unclear, but it looks like they may help to protect us against diseases, including cancer: a kind of fetal insurance policy that boosts the chances of Mom surviving long enough to support her offspring into adulthood.

This transfer of fetal cells starts from around four to six weeks of pregnancy (before many women even realize they're pregnant) and continues until birth. Even though these cells are foreign and should trigger an immune reaction in the mother, they don't appear to—although some have suggested that as well as protecting Mom against disease, they may occasionally contribute to autoimmune diseases such as rheumatoid arthritis or lupus.

Fetal cells have been recovered from the livers of women with hepatitis C, suggesting that these cells may have lodged there and transformed into liver cells to help patch up the damage caused by the disease. Meanwhile, women with breast and other cancers seem to have fewer fetal cells in their blood than healthy women, hinting that this fetal repair kit may help protect women against the disease—possibly by helping the immune system to identify and destroy cancer cells before they take hold. In addition, animal studies have shown that fetal cells can travel into the brain and mature into different cell types, including neurons (which transmit electrical signals throughout the brain) and the cells that nurture and support them.

It works in reverse, too. Babies get a transfusion of their mother's cells during pregnancy, and these, too, can stick around for years. There's even evidence that these maternal cells may help baby girls to have a successful pregnancy of their own once they grow up. Preeclampsia is a serious complication of pregnancy affecting 6 to 8 percent of women and is characterized by high blood pressure and protein in the urine. Its exact cause is unknown, but one theory is that it is triggered by the mother's immune system overresponding to the pregnancy. Hilary Gammill and her colleagues at the Fred Hutchinson Cancer Research Center in Seattle recently investigated how a woman's risk of preeclampsia related to the number of maternal cells she harbored.

In general, the number of these maternal cells increased as pregnancy progressed, suggesting that an existing population of maternal cells was being either expanded or mobilized from somewhere in the body. Whereas around 30 percent of healthy women had detectable levels of maternal cells in their blood by the third trimester, no such cells could be found in the women with preeclampsia, hinting that the maternal cells may be having some kind of protective effect. One possibility is that they may help train a woman's immune system to be more tolerant of cells from the fetus. In other words, Grandma may be indirectly helping to safeguard the survival of her family long after her own body has ceased to bear children.

THREE

BABIES

Portrait of a Newborn

. 76 .
Does birth distress the baby?

It was Sigmund Freud who first hypothesized that all anxiety could be traced back to the original trauma of being born. You could certainly imagine that birth would be a distressing event. You go from spending nine months floating in a warm cocoon to suddenly being rocked and squeezed by muscular contractions that grow increasingly violent until you find yourself being pushed down a narrow tube with such force that the bones of your skull begin to overlap. Scientists have calculated that birth exerts the equivalent of 4.4 pounds of pressure on every centimeter of the head, which sounds pretty painful.

Since none of us remembers being born and newborn babies can't speak, it's impossible to know what newborns think of the experience, but they seem to tolerate it relatively well. Recent studies have shown that newborns have high levels of stress hormones called catecholamines in their blood, which may exert a sedative effect, as well as high levels of the natural painkiller beta-endorphin, which blocks pain signals in the brain. Newborns who have endured a vaginal birth also seem to be less sensitive to pain than babies born by C-section—at least until the effects of these natural drugs wear off. Many newborns are given a routine injection of vitamin K shortly after birth, which usually prompts them to screw up their faces and scream. But when Swedish researchers compared how babies born vaginally and by C-section reacted to these injections, and then to a cold spoon being pressed against their bellies, they recorded less extreme reactions in those who had been through a vaginal birth. The heart rate of babies delivered vaginally also remained relatively stable compared to those of babies born by C-section, which shot up in response to the pain.

It's not only endorphins that might blunt pain during birth. Oxytocin is also released in large quantities during labor, and some of it will find its way across the placenta and into the baby. French researchers recently tested how newborn and two-day-old rat pups responded to painful stimuli and found that the newborns had far higher pain thresholds than the older rat pups. When newborn rats were given drugs that blocked the action of oxytocin, they became more responsive to pain.

Still other studies suggest that oxytocin temporarily dampens a baby's brain activity immediately before birth by inhibiting the ability of nerve cells to communicate with one another. As well as reducing the transmission of pain signals, this would have the added advantage of reducing the brain's energy and oxygen needs at precisely the same time as its supply of oxygen is most likely to be disrupted: as the baby is squeezed through the birth canal.

All this should provide comfort for parents whose baby needs additional help to be delivered, be it through the use of forceps that squeeze the head even further, or through a vacuum applied to the top of the head that pulls the baby out. The chances are they're dosed up on natural painkillers, so it won't be too traumatic.

. 77 .
Why do newborns look like their dads?

It's very unfair. Women spend nine months being pregnant and have the difficult job of pushing the baby out and then feeding it, only to be told constantly: "Ooooh! She looks just like her dad."

The jury is out on whether the resemblance between a baby and its father is real or imaginary. One famous paper published in *Nature* in 1995 found there was a link. Nicholas Christenfeld and Emily Hill of the University of California in San Diego gathered photos of twenty-four people when they were one, ten, and twenty years of age. They then showed the photos to 122 volunteers and asked them to match the same children at different ages, which they were very good at. But when photos of three possible parents were introduced, things became interesting. Generally, the volunteers found it difficult to match children to either parent, except when it came to matching pictures of one-year-olds to their dads (they couldn't match one-year-olds to their moms, though). Here, they guessed right 50 percent of the time, compared to the 33 percent one would expect if they were taking a random guess.

This is what evolutionary psychology would predict: Babies who look more like their dads are less likely to be rejected and therefore are more likely to survive. Given that up to 10 percent of fathers are thought to be cuckolds, it would be a neat trick. However, disgruntled moms may take comfort from several later studies that contradict this. In one, Robert French of INSERM in France and Serge Brédart of the University of Liège in Belgium tried to replicate the original study using photos of one-, three- and five-year-old children and found that people were able to guess the mothers and fathers equally well.

. 78 .
What do newborns know?

Out pops a newborn baby, bleary-eyed and baffled as it tries to make sense of its surroundings. Most people assume that newborn babies are blank slates born with no knowledge of the wider world. What could they know? They've never seen any of this before.

But babies seem to come with a certain wisdom built in. Some of it may be genetically hardwired, while some of it may have been accrued through the baby's time in the warm, dimly lit uterus, where it has been able to see, hear, feel, and taste for several months.

Some people may wonder how you go about testing what young babies know and feel, as they obviously can't tell us with words. There are a few techniques that researchers use, which, although less than perfect, may give some indication of what's going on inside those tiny heads. One is tracking the movement of a baby's eyes or head, as newborns tend to be attracted to interesting sights and sounds—particularly if they haven't seen something before. They will also turn their head to fixate on something they like, such as their mom's face. Another way of tuning in to a baby's preference is by using a device that allows them to choose between two different stimuli (such as their mother's and a stranger's voice) through the intensity of their sucking. Babies can control the rate and pressure at which they suck, even when they're not hungry, so they can be taught to turn on a certain stimulus if they suck hard enough.

Researchers can also measure a baby's emotions by looking at its facial expressions or the intensity of its cries, especially if these are combined with physiological measurements, such as its heart rate, or the release of stress hormones, such as cortisol and adrenaline.

Here's a guide to the seven pillars of innate baby wisdom. Newborn babies already understand:

Who their mother is

Babies seem to recognize their mother's voice and possibly her smell from birth, having spent months becoming accustomed to them both. Babies begin to hear during the second trimester, and though the sounds of the outside world will be distorted by the time they reach the tender ears, many do get through. Particularly prominent will be Mom's voice, as its vibrations are transmitted through her bones to the uterus.

In the 1980s, a psychologist named Anthony James DeCasper showed that babies only a couple of hours old already knew the sound of their mother's voice. He tested this by creating a feeding contraption that enabled babies to hear a recording of their mother's voice or a stranger's reading Dr. Seuss's *And to Think That I Saw It on Mulberry Street*. Judging by how hard they sucked, the newborns had a stronger preference for their mother's voice, despite being just a few hours old. Using the same contraption, DeCasper showed that babies who had been read Dr. Seuss's *The Cat in the Hat* during pregnancy preferred to listen to it over an unfamiliar story. Although they probably don't recognize the words, it's possible that they tune in to the rhythms and intonations.

Newborns also seem to be attracted to their mother's smell. In a separate study, thirty newborn babies were each placed on their mother's chest within minutes of birth; before this happened, one of the mother's breasts was washed with unscented soap in order to remove its natural odor. Twenty-two of the babies showed a clear preference for suckling the unwashed breast rather than the clean one. Another study found that five-day-old babies presented with either a clean cotton pad or one that had been worn next to their mother's breast turned to and started wriggling toward the pad that smelled of their mother (see 83: "Does skin-to-skin contact really soothe my baby?").

Knowing Mom's voice and smell must be a great source of comfort to a newborn thrust into an otherwise unfamiliar world, and within a couple of hours, it recognize's her face as well. Although babies seem to be born with an innate appreciation of the human face (see page 136), several studies have found that they rapidly start to discriminate between different faces. In a study conducted at Glasgow Hospital in Scotland during the late 1980s, two new moms with similar hair and skin color were seated next to each other behind a clear plastic screen, to mask their smell. Their babies were then brought into the room one by one and held thirty centimeters from the women's faces. An independent observer watched as the babies turned their head from one woman to the other before eventually fixating upon one of them. Despite poor eyesight and being only between twelve hours and four days old, the babies knew who their mother was and turned to gaze at her with adoration.

What it is to be human

For at least a few weeks before birth, a baby will have had the opportunity to see its surroundings, particularly on a hot summer's day, when its mom may have exposed her heavily pregnant belly to the sun, allowing more light to penetrate through the layers of skin, fat, and muscle and into the uterus.

What a baby hasn't seen is a human face, yet from the moment of birth, newborns seem hardwired to know that a triangular pattern of blobs roughly corresponding to the position of the eyes and mouth has special significance.

Studies have shown consistently that newborn babies will turn their heads to look at face-shaped patterns over random patterns, and normal faces over faces where the position of the features has been distorted. They'll also spend longer looking at them. Even nine-minute-old babies are more likely to turn their head and follow a face-like pattern over a pattern containing the same features scrambled into a different arrangement. It's as if they're born with a built-in face detector.

They also seem to understand that open eyes have some special significance. At Addenbrookes Hospital in Cambridge, UK, researchers took 105 babies who were only a couple of hours old and showed them two pictures: one of a woman with her eyes closed, the other of the same woman with her eyes open. The babies spent significantly longer looking at the picture of the woman with open eyes.

Stranger still, newborns seem capable of relating their own facial features to those of another person. In a separate study, Andrew Meltzoff of the University of Washington filmed newborns while an adult opened his mouth or stuck his tongue out at them; a third person (who couldn't see the faces the adult was pulling) rated the expressions the babies made. Time after time, these tiny babies appeared to mimic the facial expressions of the adult. This is no mean feat, considering the babies needed not only to recognize that the object in front of them was a face and that the moist pink appendage sticking out at them related to their tongue; they also required the coordination to stick out their own tongue in response.

Within a few days, newborns seem capable of discriminating between different types of facial expression. If you show babies pictures of happy or fearful faces, they will spend longer looking at happy faces—although this could be because the predominant expression of the faces they have seen during their first few days are the adoring and happy faces of their parents, rather than because of some kind of innate desire to look on the brighter side of life.

Numbers

It will be some time before your baby can count to ten, but babies are born with an appreciation of numbers as abstract concepts. This means they understand that seven objects are different from two objects, regardless of what those objects are. Until recently, people assumed that a concept of numbers was something you learned, not something you were born with.

One way of testing this is to see if babies can make the link between seven objects that they see and seven sounds that they can hear. Véronique Izard and her colleagues at Harvard University took sixteen babies aged seven hours to a hundred hours and played them a tape of spoken syllables repeated a set number of times—for example, "ba ba ba ba ba"—while showing them collections of circles or squares on a screen. Sometimes the number of objects tallied with the number of sounds, and other times it didn't, but the babies seemed to spot when they matched and spent significantly longer looking at the screen.

How do they do it? Other recent studies in both animals and humans have suggested that the brain contains specialized cells called accumulator neurons that fire in response to collections of objects—so, the more things you see, the more cells fire.

Movement and distance

Imagine being cast into the big wide world for the first time. Suddenly, you go from seeing very little to being bombarded with lights, sights, and movement. But newborns come equipped with some ideas about what they should pay attention to if they're to make sense of the world. For one thing, they know that movement is important. Move a toy back and forth in front of a newborn's face, and she will follow it with her eyes. Studies that tracked the movement of newborns' eyes have found that newborns pay more attention to the edges of objects rather than their interiors.

However, babies know that if objects are passing their eyes as if they are moving forward, then their bodies should be moving forward, too. Have you ever had the sensation when you're sitting on a train and the train next to you begins to move? For a moment, you feel as if your train is the one that's moving; if you're standing, you may lurch forward yourself. Something similar happens if you sit a newborn in a room where the walls can move independently of the floor. Even though the baby is sitting still, if the walls begin to move toward them, its head instinctively moves backward.

Similarly (and possibly because of this), newborns also understand that objects should get bigger as they move closer to them—something called size constancy. Imagine you're shown a cube, then you're shown the same cube twice as far away. You'd probably realize it was the same cube, even though it was only half the size of the original one. So do newborn babies. Alan Slater and his colleagues at the University of Exeter, UK, took two-day-old babies and showed them variations of either a small or large cube at different distances from their eyes. The babies spent longer looking at the odd cube than the cubes that fitted the pattern, suggesting that they appreciated there was something wrong.

The fundamentals of language

Although babies don't speak their first meaningful words until around the age of one, a newborn already has some appreciation of what makes his or her native language unique. Just days after birth, babies can tell the difference between different languages, even if the two languages are spoken by the same person.

They also seem to be particularly attuned to tones of voice conveying happy emotions. In one study, newborn babies were played recordings of the same passage of script read in a happy, sad, angry, or neutral voice. The newborns were more likely to open their eyes and look as if they were paying attention when they heard the happy voice, compared to when the same passage was read in the other tones of voice. However, this happened only when the speaker used the baby's native language. If the child of an English-speaking mother heard a happy-sounding Spanish woman, it paid little attention to her. One possible explanation is that fetuses can detect physical signs related to different emotional states—such as anger prompting an increase in breathing, heart rate, and muscle tension—and they learn to associate these states with particular sounds.

Newborns seem to cry in a melody befitting their native tongue. A recent study of sixty French and German newborns found differences in the intonation patterns of their cries. Whereas the wails of French babies start low and end on a high note, German babies cry in a falling melody—patterns that chime with the intonation patterns of adult speakers of these languages. Since crying may be the only sound newborn babies know how to make, it may sometimes represent their first attempt at communication, the researchers suggest. At any rate, it suggests they have been paying attention to language during pregnancy.

Empathy (or the difference between themselves and others)

Okay, it'll be several years before your child truly grasps the notion that other people have thoughts and feelings of their own (see 127: "When do babies develop a sense of themselves as individuals?"), but even newborns react to the emotions of others. Have you ever noticed how, if one baby starts crying, it sets off every other baby in the room? They're not just responding to loud noise.

Back in the 1970s, researchers found that if they played a newborn a recording of other babies crying, then it started crying as well. When they did the same thing with recordings of equally loud and intense nonhuman sounds, the babies cried less. So babies seem to know they're babies and get upset when others are upset. In a later study, Italian researchers played newborn babies recordings of their own cries and the cries of other babies to see how they responded. The babies showed more visible signs of distress, such as knitting their eyebrows together, screwing up their eyes, and grimacing, when they heard the other babies cry, compared to when they heard their own cries, suggesting that they could discriminate between the two. Some people have interpreted this as evidence that the early roots of empathy are present at birth, while others believe it may be a primitive response to a distress call—similar to the way birds and other animals signal to each other when a predator is approaching.

By the age of eighteen months, most babies have begun to grasp the concept that other people have different likes and dislikes than they do, and they will react accordingly. For example, if you show babies a bowl of crackers and a bowl of broccoli, most infants will make a beeline for the crackers; but if you make a face to show that you love broccoli and pull a disgusted face at the crackers, an eighteen-month-old will generally offer you some broccoli.

However, true empathy, when you notice someone else's distress and are moved to do something to make it better, doesn't develop until around the age of two. In the book *The Scientist in the Crib,* developmental psychologist Alison Gopnik describes her son's reaction when she came back from a particularly tough day at the lab to find the chicken legs that she'd planned to cook for dinner still frozen. Like any frazzled mom, she broke down in tears on the sofa. Upon seeing this, her son, who was approaching the age of two, looked thoughtful and then ran to the bathroom and came back with a large box of bandages, which he proceeded to stick all over her to try to make her better. I have a similar story about my daughter, Matilda, when she was twenty-two months old and had been to the doctor's for shots. The next day, I returned home from work heavily pregnant, utterly exhausted, and with pains in my belly, and slumped on the sofa. Matilda climbed on to my lap and patted the bandage on her arm. With a genuine expression of concern etched across her little face, she patted her arm and told me: "Mummy need medicine from doctor."

A natural sense of rhythm/music

If you're going to be a dancer or a musician, you need to sense the beat. And a baby's ears seem to be tuned to detect rhythm from the moment it is born.

Since babies can't exactly click their fingers in time with a tune, István Winkler and his colleagues at the Hungarian Academy of Sciences in Budapest monitored their brain activity instead. If an adult is played a regular rhythm and that rhythm is disrupted, then the brain produces a characteristic signature that can be detected with an EEG cap using tiny sensors to pick up electrical signals.

To see if newborn babies showed the same response, Winkler played them variations of a rock rhythm involving a snare drum, a bass drum, and a high-hat cymbal. When beats that were unimportant to the overall rhythm were omitted, the babies showed no response, but when the critical downbeat was absent, the babies' brains detected this disruption to the rhythm.

Researchers had suggested previously that babies learn rhythm as a result of being rocked by their parents, but Winkler's study suggests that a sense of rhythm may be innate. Another possibility is that the fetus learns about rhythm in the uterus by listening to its mother's heartbeat and the sounds that filter in from the outside world. An appreciation of rhythm isn't important just for music; it may also help babies to learn about language by disentangling the speech patterns that convey certain emotions or set some languages apart from others. Similar studies looking at babies' brain activity have suggested that newborns can detect differences in pitch and whether a series of notes is rising or falling in scale.

. 79 .
How much can newborns see?

Open most baby books and you'll read that newborns can focus only on objects twelve inches in front of them, which, coincidentally, is often the distance they're held away from the mother's face. This is a myth born out of a scientific paper published in the 1960s, the conclusions of which have since been overturned several times.

Actually, newborns can focus on objects at any distance, but they're not very good at it because the brain has not yet fine-tuned the connections that allow it to adjust the thickness of the lens and bring things into sharp focus. It's a bit like letting a very clumsy person loose with a manual-focus camera—they'll often over- or undershoot, and the image will come out blurred.

Very young babies sometimes give the impression that they are focusing on nearby objects because they struggle to coordinate the movements of the left and right eyes and keep them pointing in the same direction, which means they can look slightly cross-eyed. Their attention also tends to be drawn to objects close at hand, such as Mom's eyes, mouth, nipples, and their own hands. "Because they may not yet have good control of eye coordination, when they try to focus on close objects, they can overconverge their eyes, making it appear to us that they are focused very, very close indeed," adds Russell Hamer, an affiliate scientist at the Smith-Kettlewell Eye Research Institute in San Francisco. Newborns also struggle to integrate the input from both eyes to produce a 3-D picture, so, for the first few months, they see the world in flat 2-D.

Another reason why even nearby objects will appear grainy to a newborn baby is that other visual areas are not fully developed. These include the retina—the area at the back of the eye on which images are focused—

and regions of the brain that interpret these images. For example, an area in the middle of the retina called the fovea is important for seeing details, but it takes many months before enough receptor cells (called cones) have developed and are mature enough to signal very fine details to the brain.

When Hamer and his colleagues measured newborns' visual acuity, or their ability to see details, they discovered that it is around six times poorer than that of adults. To put it another way, if you think of those eye charts used by opticians to test your eyesight, the only letter that newborns would be able to make out clearly would be the "E" on the top line. By four months of age, this aspect of eyesight is much better, but it's not until eight to twelve months that babies' eyesight approaches adult standards. By three years or so, they achieve 20/20 vision.

That's not to say that babies can't see an awful lot. Even if it can make out only that "E" on the eye chart, a newborn baby can see two flies sitting on a white wall from about 2.3 meters, Dad's smile from about 9 meters, or a 70-meter Boeing 747 from over ten miles.

"A young infant's acuity is good enough to see most of the things that are important to him or her," says Hamer. "Even a newborn infant held in your arms can easily see your eyes, your lips and smile, your nose. They can also see their own hands, fingers, feet, and toes."

There are other differences between how babies see the world and how most adults do. The fovea is important for color vision, so as well as the world appearing blurry, newborn babies can't perceive color properly until they're around four months old—although one study suggests that they are able to tell the difference between red and green from as young as two weeks. Difficulties may start to creep in once they try to distinguish between subtle shades such as light blue and turquoise.

New parents are told they need to buy toys with large, high-contrast black-and-white patterns so their baby can see them and to stimulate visual development, but modern research suggests that this isn't correct. This was based on the belief that babies had little or no color vision (which isn't true) and that their sensitivity to low contrasts was limited. However, studies have shown that, for reasonably large patterns, the visual areas of even very young infants' brains can respond to low contrasts, and by nine weeks, babies are only two times less sensitive to contrast than adults. "By about two months of age, your baby is capable of perceiving almost all of the subtle shadings that make our visual world so rich, textured, and interesting: shadings in clouds, shadows that are unique to your face; they can even see a white teddy bear on a white couch," says Hamer.

. 80 .
Why do newborns have blue eyes?

Eye color is inherited from your parents and is determined by the amount of a pigment called melanin that you produce. People who don't produce much melanin have blue or gray eyes, while those who produce lots of melanin have brown eyes.

At birth, very little melanin is being produced, regardless of the genes you have inherited. This is why most babies' eyes appear blue or blue-gray. As babies' eyes are exposed to light, production of melanin is ramped up, so if babies are genetically programmed to produce lots of melanin, their eye color will begin to change as the months go by. A baby's eye color usually settles down by around the age of six months and is unlikely to change much afterward.

. 81 .
How do babies go from breathing nothing to breathing air?

A baby's body undergoes several massive changes in the minutes and hours after birth. Before birth, the baby has "breathed" by exchanging oxygen and carbon dioxide with its mother's blood via the placenta. Now it needs to switch to breathing through its lungs, but in the womb, these are deflated and filled with amniotic fluid—hardly ideal for breathing air. Healthy babies have about eight ounces of fluid in their lungs, which they need to get rid of in order to breathe. Around a third is squeezed out as a result of contractions and being pushed through the birth canal during labor, which compresses the chest. Labor also triggers the production of chemicals called catecholamines, which tell the lungs to start absorbing fluid. Finally, as the baby's chest emerges from its mother's body, it naturally expands, drawing in air. This displaces the remaining fluid from the lungs, much as blowing through a straw into a full glass of water will cause some of the water to be pushed out of the glass and onto the table.

What about babies delivered by planned C-section? Their mothers don't go through labor, so how does the baby know to start breathing? Part of the answer lies in the clamping of the umbilical cord, which stops the flow of oxygen and triggers a reflex that causes the baby to gasp for air, inflating the lungs and displacing some of the fluid. But most babies delivered by C-section will start breathing before the cord is clamped, so there must be other mechanisms at work. The physical act of removing the baby from the uterus causes the uterus to contract, and this squeezes the placenta and reduces the flow of the baby's blood into it. These contractions also trigger the placenta to start peeling away from the wall of the uterus (as happens in a natural birth). Studies in animals have suggested that exposing the nose to oxygen in the air is enough to initiate breathing, while being brought from the warmth of the mother's body into a cold operating room also seems to stimulate this reflex.

For about four months before birth, the baby's lungs have been manufacturing a substance called surfactant, which helps repel water from the lining of the lungs and enables them to inflate and take up oxygen. Babies born by C-section may still have some fluid in the lungs, so they may be watched for any signs of breathing difficulties.

As the lungs fill with air, this activates another big change in the baby. Before birth, very little blood is pumped from the heart to the lungs, whereas in adults, the entire right side of the heart is devoted to this purpose—sending the deoxygenated blood it receives to the lungs to be loaded up with oxygen, which then reenters the left side of the heart to be pumped back out to the rest of the body. Before birth, there is a hole between the right and left sides of the heart that largely cuts out the lungs from the circulation. But as the lungs fill with air, this fundamentally changes their structure and makes it far easier to pump blood through them. Because of this, the blood pressure in some of the vessels feeding the heart changes, which prompts a one-way flap of tissue to slam shut over the hole that previously allowed blood to pass from the right to the left side of the heart. The baby's heart and lungs are now plumbed in to work like an adult's.

The tiny baby breathes a sigh of relief. Its transition to life outside the womb is complete.

. 82 .
Why do newborn babies smell so good?

There's something about that milky newborn smell that intoxicates parents. Many admit to spending hours inhaling their baby's odor. Shortly after the birth of her twins, Emme and Max, Jennifer Lopez allegedly told her fragrance experts that she'd like her new perfume, Live, to smell like the top of a baby's head.

It's not just in our imagination. Several studies have shown that women can pick out the scent of their baby from other babies within a few days of birth, while other research has shown that new moms are more attracted to the smell of newborn infants than are non-moms.

In one study, Alison Fleming and her colleagues at the University of Toronto asked women to rate the smell of unfamiliar babies' T-shirts on a scale of attractiveness. They found that new moms rated the smells as more delicious than did non-mothers or the mothers of slightly older babies, so there may be something about being a new mom that makes you more tuned into that new-baby smell. Indeed, in a later study, Fleming's team found that moms with higher levels of cortisol—a hormone that has been linked to other aspects of maternal instinct (see 31: "Are some women naturally more maternal than others?")—were more drawn to baby odors and better at recognizing their own baby's smell than women with lower levels of cortisol.

"We also tested fathers, and they, too, like the odors of babies," says Fleming. What's more, parents' attraction to these baby body odors seems to increase, the more time they spend with their child, and their ability to recognize their own baby's smell also seems to improve with experience.

Although we don't know precisely where these smelly signals are coming from, we can hazard a guess. Small oil-producing glands—sebaceous glands—are found all over the body, but especially on the head and face, and these tend to be particularly active in newborn babies. Sweat-producing eccrine glands are present in high numbers on the heads of newborns, and secretions from both these glands serve as nutrients for bacteria—whose action is a key factor in the production of body odors, says Richard Porter, an expert in human smell at the French National Centre for Scientific Research in Nouzilly. In Fleming's study, the clean T-shirts were wiped over the babies' heads and bodies before they were given to the moms to sniff. Body odor can be influenced by what you eat, so breast-feeding (which is known to affect how babies' diapers smell) may contribute to that delicious new-baby smell. This may explain why babies stop smelling so unique once they start eating solid food at around the age of six months.

What's more, body odor has a strong inherited component. "Mothers may also be able to detect a similarity between the baby's odor and the smell of other family members, such as the infant's father or older siblings," says Porter. Other studies have shown that people can match parents to their children on the basis of their smell, while sniffer dogs have difficulty discriminating between identical twins who share the same genes.

. 83 .
Does skin-to-skin contact really soothe my baby?

What new mom doesn't dream of the moment her baby will be placed, sticky and warm, on her naked chest? But does the baby know or care what happens to it during those first crucial moments in the outside world? Although it may sound like a fluffy, new age, feel-good kind of thing, skin-to-skin contact has been surprisingly well studied by scientists, and the general consensus is that it really does make a difference to the baby's well-being.

Place a newborn baby on its mother's bare chest, and a few interesting things will start to happen. First, the baby begins to make sucking and rooting gestures with its mouth; then its arms will make crawling movements, and its legs will start to push against the skin as it slowly inches its way toward the breasts. A recent review of thirty studies looking at the effect of skin-to-skin contact found that babies who received early skin-to-skin contact with their mothers during the first few hours after birth were more likely to breast-feed, and breast-fed for an average of forty-three days longer than babies who didn't receive such contact. They also cried less and were warmer in the twenty-four hours after birth; their heart rate and breathing rate were around three beats and breaths per minute slower; and their blood-sugar levels were more stable than those of babies who didn't receive skin-to-skin contact.

That babies who receive skin-to-skin contact are warmer doesn't seem to be just down to the transfer of heat from their mother's skin. A recent study found that some babies who were held to the skin within two hours of birth still had warmer feet, twenty-three hours later, than babies who spent their first hours in a crib. One explanation is that being held close to Mom reverses some of the effects of stress caused by the birth. Stress tends to divert blood flow away from extremities such as the feet, which would make them colder, and causes more of the baby's energy reserves to be used up, which might help to explain why babies who don't receive early skin-to-skin contact have lower blood-sugar levels.

Although it's not particularly surprising that newborns who are separated from their mothers cry more, what's interesting is that the type of cry they make is remarkably similar to a specific distress call made by other newborn mammals. One study that looked at crying in newborns found that it was virtually absent in babies in close contact with their moms, while those in cribs tended to cry in short pulses of seven to forty-two seconds, separated by silent periods. When the researchers analyzed recordings of these cries, they found that the pattern was very similar in different babies, and it stopped as soon as they were united with their mothers. It was also distinct from other types of cry, such as those signaling hunger or pain.

One reason why babies might be separated from their mothers after birth is to give women some time to rest and recuperate, but if it's peace and quiet you're after, then it seems that the best solution may be to hold the baby close to you—at least in these very early days.

Skin-to-skin contact may have other benefits for Mom. The pushing movements the baby makes with its legs stimulate the uterus to contract, helping to seal off the flow of blood as the placenta begins to peel away from the uterus and is delivered. Breast tissue also becomes profoundly sensitive to touch just before birth, and any contact with it seems to trigger a surge of oxytocin, a hormone well known to promote social bonding. Previous studies in other mammals have suggested that newborns deliberately knead or paw the udders, and this stimulates the production of both oxytocin and milk.

Video recordings of newborn babies placed on their mother's naked chest suggest that they may do something similar. Around six minutes after birth, a newborn baby opens its eyes and starts to look around. Five minutes later, its hands, which were initially open and relaxed, begin to perform rhythmic, massage-like "milking" movements on its mother's breast, which increase in frequency over the coming hour. Twenty minutes after birth, the baby begins to root or make sucking motions with its mouth, and shortly afterward, it begins to touch its mom's nipple, which becomes more erect as a result. Now the baby begins to lick the nipple, all the while continuing to massage its mother's breast. Finally, around eighty minutes after the birth, the newborn baby puts the nipple in its mouth and begins to suck.

The researchers who recorded these sequences took blood samples from the mothers at regular intervals and found that their levels of oxytocin rose as the frequency of the baby's hand movements increased. Besides promoting bonding between Mom and baby, this may also help explain why early skin-to-skin contact is linked to higher rates of breast-feeding. Many researchers think that the first hours after birth represent a critical period in which the connections between breast stimulation and the brain become reinforced. Others have noticed that levels of feel-good chemicals in the blood (called endorphins) double during breast-feeding, which might also promote bonding.

So what should parents do if Mom is unable to have early skin-to-skin contact with her baby, perhaps because of a medical emergency? Moms who have to be separated from their baby for prolonged periods can try massaging their breasts to mimic the baby's actions. Getting Dad to strip off and cuddle the baby may also have some effect (and I bet most dads would relish the chance to bond with their newborn). In 2007, Swedish researchers set out to investigate how babies respond to immediate skin-to-skin contact with their dads when their mothers were unable to hold them. It was a small study of twenty-nine babies, around half of whom had immediate skin-to-skin contact with their dads, while the rest were placed in cribs beside them. Within fifteen minutes, the babies held by their dads had dramatically reduced their crying, and after sixty minutes, they had entered a calm and drowsy state, while the babies lying in cribs took around 110 minutes to reach the same state.

Putting the baby on Dad's chest may also kick-start his paternal instinct: Men release oxytocin in response to cuddling and interacting with their babies, and the more oxytocin they release, the more time they seem to want to spend with them (see 32: "Do men change when they become dads?").

. 84 .
How do newborns know to seek the nipple for food?

Babies are born with an acute sense of smell, and early studies hint that they may use this to guide them toward their one and only food source: milk. In 2001, researchers conducted a fascinating experiment. Twenty-one newborns ranging from thirty-six hours to four days old were placed on to a warm bed, and either a clean cotton pad or one that their mothers had been wearing next to their breast for several hours was put in front of them, just out of reach. Using their legs to propel them forward, the babies began to inch their way toward the pads. Within three minutes, eighteen of the babies had inched toward the pad that smelled of the breast, compared to just three of the babies when they were given the control pad to examine.

Many women may notice that the area surrounding their nipples becomes increasingly bumpy during pregnancy, and that these bumps, called Montgomery's tubercles, sometimes secrete an oily fluid. It was previously assumed that this fluid helped to keep the nipple lubricated, but Benoist Schaal and his colleagues at the National Centre for Scientific Research in Dijon, France, recently found that it may also help guide the baby to the breast. When they collected these secretions and exposed three-day-old babies to them, they found that the babies made more sucking and licking movements than when they smelled other scents, such as sweat or breast milk. Schaal also found that women with more than nine glands per breast started lactating around ten hours sooner than women with fewer glands, while their babies also fed more frequently and gained weight more quickly. It's not only babies who may be sensitive to these odors. Another recent study found that smells associated with breast-feeding may put women in the mood for sex. Breast-feeding women were asked to wear cotton pads next to their breasts and in their armpits for eight hours. A separate group of women were then given pads worn by the lactating women or unscented pads and asked to wipe them over their upper lip each morning and evening for three months, as well as keeping a diary of their sex lives and levels of sexual desire.

The women given pads worn by breast-feeding women experienced an increase in sexual desire and sexual fantasies, particularly during the second half of their menstrual cycle, when desire usually falls. Whether the chemicals responsible for this aphrodisiac effect are the same as those that newborns use to find the breast is unclear—neither has anyone tested whether men get similarly aroused by the smell of female breasts—but you might want to think more carefully about how you dispose of those used breast pads in future.

. 85 .
What causes the Moro or "startle" reflex?

Your brand-new baby is lying peacefully in his or her crib when you accidentally bump against its sides. Melodramatically, the baby arches its back and flings its legs and arms out to the side with fingers spread, as if someone just poured a bucket of cold water over its head.

Babies are born with a number of reflexes—actions performed in response to a stimulus, without conscious thought—but the Moro reflex is probably the most dramatic (and amusing) of them. It is triggered if you bang something against the surface the baby is lying on, or if the baby's head drops slightly below the level of its body. Some have proposed that in our distant past the Moro reflex helped babies to survive by prompting them to cling on to and embrace their mothers if they felt as though they were falling.

Another reflex that could have played a similar role is the grasp reflex, which you can test by placing your finger in the center of a newborn's palm: It should grip tightly enough to hold even its own body weight. Back in 1891, Louis Robinson tested how long newborn infants were able to cling to a horizontal rod with both hands using the grasp reflex. After testing sixty babies under the age of one month, he concluded that most could hang on for at least ten seconds, while one plucky infant managed to hang from the rod for two minutes and thirty-five seconds before letting go.

Monkeys also have these reflexes, which supports the idea that they may have been important in our evolutionary past. The grasp reflex is even stronger in baby monkeys, which often cling to their mother's coats as they are carried around; tests have shown that they can hang one-handed from a horizontal rod for between seven and thirty-three minutes.

Although apes and monkeys also possess the Moro reflex, this doesn't necessarily protect them against falls. One problem is that the main feature of the Moro reflex is the throwing out of the arms, rather than clinging on and embracing something—although neither babies nor monkeys produce the Moro reflex if they are grasping something at the time.

A group of Japanese researchers recently proposed that, rather than using the Moro reflex to break its fall, a baby may use it to catch its mother's attention if she starts to drop it. If a baby flings out its arms dramatically, Mom would immediately grab on it and prevent its fall.

There are several other interesting reflexes you might want to look out for:

Rooting reflex

If you stroke your baby's cheek, it should start to turn toward your finger; this may help babies to find the nipple. This reflex disappears after about three months.

Tonic neck reflex

If you turn your baby's head to one side while he's awake and lying on his back, he should extend the same arm in front of his eyes and flex his other arm; this might help prepare the baby for reaching. The reflex disappears after about four months.

Stepping reflex

If you hold your baby under his arms with his feet touching the floor, he should start lifting his legs in a stepping motion; this may help prepare babies for walking. The reflex disappears after around two months.

Babinski reflex

If you stroke the sole of your baby's foot from toe to heel, you will probably see his toes spread out and curl as the foot curls in; the purpose of this reflex is unknown. It disappears at eight to twelve months.

Swimming reflex

Dunk a baby facedown into a pool of water, and he'll instinctively hold his breath, paddle, and kick in a swimming motion. Take care with this one, as a baby may still swallow large amounts of water. The reflex may have evolved to help babies survive if they fall into water, but it disappears at four to six months.

Baby Bodies

. 86 .
Are baby growth charts accurate?

It's a moment many moms come to dread: going to the well-child clinic to get the baby weighed and being told he isn't growing fast enough, or that he's surprisingly big for his age (even though he looks and seems perfectly healthy).

In the U.S., babies are usually weighed and measured at each well-child visit; these measurements will be checked against standard growth charts, which tell you roughly how your baby compares to others of the same age. Seven lines snake their way across traditional U.S. growth charts, each representing a "percentile" above or below the average. If your baby's weight lies on the fifth centile, this means that for every one hundred healthy babies of the same age, five would be expected to weigh less and ninety-five would weigh more.

Growth charts can be a great source of anxiety for new parents, particularly as babies can jump up and down centiles within a matter of weeks. My daughter was on the twenty-fifth centile for the first four weeks and then slipped down to the ninth centile before starting to climb up toward the fiftieth. Each time I was told not to worry, with the caveat that if she continued on the same trajectory, it might be time to worry.

More experienced moms informed me that growth charts are inaccurate because they're based on measurements of bottle-fed babies, who tend to be heavier, although the truth is that this depends on the country you live in and the charts being used. But the argument is fast becoming redundant, because the U.S. and many other countries recently replaced their old charts with growth charts provided by the World Health Organization (WHO), which are based on data from exclusively breast-fed babies.

You'll know if the chart your doctor is using is one of the new WHO charts because there are just five lines, and the fiftieth centile (the middle line) is no longer emphasized in bold as it was on the older charts, so parents feel less that this is the ideal weight that all babies should be striving to attain.

The WHO introduced the new charts in 2006 after collecting data from babies born in six different countries. Because exclusive breast-feeding is now considered the gold standard by the WHO and many other health organizations, the idea behind the charts was to describe growth as it should occur under optimum conditions rather than as it occurs in the general population.

However, the introduction of the new charts has not been entirely without controversy. Compared with existing growth charts from the U.S. and the Netherlands, and a multinational growth chart representing other European countries, babies measured against the WHO charts are judged to be heavier during the first six months of life and lighter between six and twenty-four months of age. In other words, a four-month-old baby previously classified as healthy might now be classified as underweight, while a twelve-month-old previously thought to be a normal weight might now be judged as overweight.

This has come as a surprise to many, as these previous charts included some bottle-fed babies, who are generally assumed to be heavier. One explanation is that the criteria used to decide which babies should be included in the WHO study were so strict that they have led to a skewed picture of what weight gain should look like in breast-fed babies. If the WHO standards really are too high, this could serve to discourage women from exclusive breast-feeding, or to give up altogether. "If the child's weight is toward the low end of the range, a mother may conclude that her milk supply is inadequate," says Ekhard Ziegler, a professor of pediatrics at the University of Iowa in Iowa City. Despite the CDC's recommendation to switch to WHO charts when assessing babies under the age of two, Ziegler says that many U.S. pediatricians continue to use the older charts, as they think they're more representative of the normal U.S. population.

Tim Cole, a statistician at the MRC Centre of Epidemiology for Child Health in London, who helped adapt the WHO charts for the UK, says the patterns aren't necessarily suspicious. Although the common perception is that bottle-fed babies are heavier, "breast-fed babies do grow rapidly to start with and then slow down," he says.

So what message should new parents take away? If even the experts can't agree on the best way of assessing a baby's weight, perhaps we should all relax and stop worrying about how our baby's growth is tracking compared to the average. So long as they're not completely off the charts, chances are they're fine.

Growth charts are supposed to reflect the fact that individual babies differ in height and build, so there's nothing wrong with your baby being in the first centile or the ninety-ninth centile. Another common misunderstanding is that regardless of how heavy a baby is, it should broadly stick to the same growth curve and not switch from one centile to another.

A baby's birth weight doesn't reflect just the weight it is genetically programmed to be but how good the mother's uterus and placenta were at supplying the baby with nutrients and how much the mother ate during pregnancy. Once the baby is born, these other factors cease to be relevant. This means that babies may lose or gain a fair amount of weight while they are finding their natural balance. "Particularly during the first year, babies cross centiles a lot," says Cole. "Generally, it has to be pretty extreme before people should start worrying about it, particularly during the first six months."

Neither should parents feel pressured into having their baby weighed every time they see a pediatrician. The American Academy of Pediatrics recommends weighing babies at three to five days, then at one month, two months, four months, six months, nine months, and twelve months. However, recent UK recommendations say that all babies should be weighed at six to eight weeks, and then only when there is parental or professional concern. Even where there is concern, babies shouldn't be weighed more than once a month before the age of six months, or every two months between six and twelve months. Weighing babies more frequently can lead to misleading results, because natural fluctuations in weight and differences between weighing scales may be greater than any overall weight gain during that period.

Weight gain also slows down as babies approach their first birthday. Finally, when it comes to really young babies, the growth charts should be thrown out altogether. Generally, the most important consideration during the first two weeks of a baby's life is not its position on a chart relative to other babies, but how its current weight compares to its birth weight. Most babies are expected to lose a bit of weight after birth, but they usually regain their birth weight by two weeks, and only 3 to 7 percent of babies lose as much as 10 percent of their birth weight. Even then, at least one study found no major medical problems among babies who lost more than 10 percent of their birth weight in the first twelve days. Unless doctors have a genuine medical concern about a baby's weight loss, parents shouldn't feel pressurized into feeding their baby supplemental milk, particularly if it could interfere with the establishment of breast-feeding.

. 87 .
Do big babies grow into big adults?

It is clear that tall parents tend to produce tall children, but factors such as putting on a lot of weight or smoking during pregnancy and gestational diabetes are known to impact on a baby's size at birth. Mothers seem to have a greater influence over a baby's growth during pregnancy than fathers, probably as a means of safeguarding against serious birth complications (see 16: "Do big parents have bigger babies?").

That said, several studies have found an association between a baby's length and weight at birth and the size it grows into as an adult. The strongest correlation seems to be for length. As a rough guide, one recent study from Denmark found that baby boys who were shorter than 18.5 inches at birth grew into men with an average height of 5 feet and 7 and a half inches, while those longer than 22 inches had an adult height of 6 feet. Unfortunately, it didn't look at baby girls' heights.

A separate study found that birth weight and length make independent contributions to the eventual size of a person. So if your newborn is both long and heavy, you may well have a future giant on your hands.

. 88 .
Why don't babies have moles?

The majority of babies are born with flawless skin, but moles and freckles will appear as they progress through childhood and adolescence, usually from the age of around six months. By the time they are adults, most will have around twelve to twenty perfectly harmless moles on their skin.

Exactly what triggers mole growth is unknown, but it is likely to be an interaction between genetic factors and sun exposure. Moles tend to appear on skin that is exposed regularly to the sun, and they usually start off as a flat, round spot that will grow evenly on both sides as the child gets older. The mole may start to grow into a raised bump, and it may get lighter or darker, but unless the mole looks itchy, bleeds, or is different from other moles, it is unlikely to be anything to worry about.

Many studies have shown that moles are more common in children with fair skin or those who are exposed to the sun, so if your child plays outside a lot, then keeping her skin covered up with clothing should reduce the number of moles that appear. How many moles a child will develop is inherited to a certain extent, so if you and your partner have a lot of moles, your baby is likely to develop more. While a few moles are nothing to worry about, having lots (more than a hundred when you're an adult) seems to put you at increased risk of skin cancer. Going on vacation to hot countries also seems to increase a child's chances of developing moles.

Around 1 percent of babies are born with a mole, which in this case is a type of birthmark. Most are harmless, but if your baby is born with a really big birthmark (over eight inches in diameter), it may be at a slightly increased risk of developing a form of skin cancer called melanoma.

. 89 .
What causes colic?

Colic is most parents' vision of hell. All babies cry, some more than others, but colic is defined as an otherwise healthy baby showing periods of intense or unexplained crying lasting over three hours a day, over three days a week, over three weeks. It tends to peak at around the age of six weeks, is usually worse in the late afternoon and evening, and often stops at the age of two to three months. Around a fifth of two-month-olds suffer from colic, and it can have serious consequences. Mothers of colicky babies are more likely to suffer from postnatal depression and more likely to give up breast-feeding, and colic occasionally prompts some to do the unthinkable: to lash out and harm their child.

For thousands of years, doctors have blamed excessive crying on problems related to digestion—indeed, the word "colic" comes from the Greek *kolikos,* which translates as "of the colon." Yet it is used as a catch-all phrase to diagnose something that may have multiple causes. Current theories include food allergy or an immature digestive system, or that it's part of normal brain development (albeit at the extreme end of the spectrum) and the idea that some babies are simply born with more difficult temperaments.

Some recent research has suggested that colic may be down to low-level inflammation of the baby's gut or painful muscle spasms (a bit like inflammatory bowel syndrome in adults). There is some evidence that herbal teas containing vervain, chamomile, fennel, licorice, or lemon balm can help colic by relaxing the muscles in the gut, but giving babies too much extra liquid can reduce the appetite for milk. A drug called Simethicone claims to reduce the surface tension of trapped air bubbles in the gut, enabling gas to be expelled more easily. Although one trial found that Simethicone reduced the number of crying attacks on days four to seven of treatment compared with placebo, the study included only twenty-six babies and provided no details on how colic was defined. Two other studies found no significant effect.

Some have suggested that colicky babies simply have "difficult" personalities, but most experts agree that this is unlikely to be a major cause of colic (though it may be a contributing factor). While there may be a link between colic and anxious parenting, it's probable that this is not a direct cause. However, parents should try to watch for early signs that their baby may be tired or hungry, as these things can make crying worse.

Many pediatricians believe that so long as babies are growing and developing normally, there is no need to treat colic, because it usually disappears with time. The trouble with this is that some babies labeled as having colic may have an underlying medical problem that could be treated, potentially ending the suffering.

In one small study of twenty-four healthy babies and nineteen babies diagnosed with colic, researchers found that up to half of those in the colic group showed evidence of feeding problems, including less rhythmic sucking and problems coordinating sucking, breathing, and swallowing. In addition, ultrasound scans revealed more evidence of gastrointestinal reflux in the colic group—something that was backed up by reports from mothers of colicky babies.

Before simply swallowing a diagnosis of colic and leaving it to run its course, you should try to eliminate some of the following causes:

Gastroesophageal reflux
Spitting up milk is extremely common among newborn babies and usually nothing to worry about. Reflux doesn't tend to cause pain, as spit-up is actually pH-neutral for two hours after a feed because milk acts as a buffer to stomach acid. However, if your colicky baby is also spitting up blood, refusing to feed, failing to gain weight, or projectile vomiting, these could be signs of more serious gastroesophageal reflux disease, and you should consult a doctor.

Infection
Infections are sometimes mistakenly labeled as colic, because they can trigger inconsolable crying. One study of 237 babies taken to a hospital because they wouldn't stop crying found that 5 percent had an underlying illness, most commonly a urinary-tract infection.

Breast-feeding problems
Failing to properly latch on to the breast can lead to excessive crying because the baby isn't getting enough milk. Classic warning signs during the first six weeks include producing fewer than six wet cloth diapers or four heavily wet disposable diapers per day, and fewer than three to four yellow stools per day (although babies do vary in how often they produce stools).

Functional lactose overload
Babies who don't feed long enough to get through the relatively watery foremilk to the creamier hindmilk can develop something called functional

lactose overload. Fat levels in milk increase as the breast-feed progresses, and this fat slows down the progress of milk through the intestines, giving it more time to be digested. But if a baby drinks only the watery foremilk, this passes through the gut too quickly, and the undigested protein then ferments in the colon. The result is frothy and explosive poops, a bloated belly, crying, and hunger. One study of seventy-seven five-week-olds found that those with colic had lower levels of a hormone that's released in response to eating a high-fat meal, suggesting that the milk they were consuming wasn't rich enough, probably because they weren't taking long enough over each feed. A different study that compared the effect of either offering one breast at each feed or both breasts for a shorter period of time found a lower incidence of colic in the babies who fed from just one breast, as well as less engorgement and mastitis among the mothers.

Food allergy

Occasionally, a baby may be allergic to something in its mother's diet; despite suggestions that moms should stop eating soy, wheat, nuts, or fish to ease their baby's discomfort, the only thing that has been linked consistently to inconsolable crying is an allergy to cows' milk. Between 5 and 15 percent of babies show symptoms suggesting they may be allergic to some of the proteins in cows' milk, but only half of these are thought to suffer from it. Key symptoms include crying, a runny nose and persistent cough, a skin rash or eczema, frequent regurgitation of milk, and diarrhea or constipation. Cutting dairy products out of your own diet for two weeks should tell you if an allergy to cows' milk is at the root of your baby's problems. If the baby is formula-feeding, you can try switching to an extensively hydrolyzed or hypoallergenic formula. According the American Academy of Pediatrics (AAP), there's no evidence supporting the use of soy-protein formula to prevent or manage colic and fussiness.

Lactose intolerance

An allergy to cows' milk is different from lactose intolerance, in which babies don't have enough of the lactase enzyme that usually breaks down a sugar found in milk called lactose. The result is too much of this sugar entering the colon, where it ferments, causing bloating and pain. Several small studies have found that babies suffering from colic have more hydrogen gas in their breath, which is a product of lactose fermentation. Likewise, a few early stud-ies have suggested that feeding babies formula treated with lactase enzyme can ease symptoms of colic in some. However, genuine lactose intolerance is pretty rare during the first year of life, and some pediatricians feel that it is being overdiagnosed. More likely is functional lactose overload or an allergy to cows' milk, although babies may develop temporary lactose intolerance as a result of damage to the gut lining caused by gastroenteritis or an allergy to cows' milk. Feeding a baby with an allergy to cows' milk a lactose-free formula may make things worse if the formula contains cows'-milk protein, as it will continue to irritate the gut.

. 90 .
What is the best way to settle a crying baby?

Anyone who has been caught in an enclosed space with a howling baby can testify to how stressful it can be. Frantic parents will try anything: rocking the baby, doing endless laps of the park with the stroller, even shelling out hundreds of pounds on cranial osteopathy, vibrating mattresses, or devices that claim to interpret a baby's cries and tell you if it is hungry, bored, sleepy, or uncomfortable. Although there will undoubtedly be babies that respond to each of these different strategies, scientists have weighed in on the issue and put some of them to the test.

One of the first strategies parents turn to is carrying the baby around with them in a sling or wrap. Studies have reached mixed conclusions about whether or not this works: Some found that it is effective so long as you start carrying before the age of six weeks, while others found no reduction in total crying. There are concerns that prolonged carrying of a baby simply teaches it how to fall asleep in its parents' arms, rather than on its own in a crib. Cer-tainly, carrying doesn't seem to be particularly helpful for babies with colic. Even in societies where babies are carried constantly by their mothers, there are babies who continue to cry inconsolably. A randomized controlled trial of sixty-six mothers who said their babies cried excessively found no difference in the duration or frequency of fussing and crying between those who rocked and soothed their babies and those who increased the amount of time they spent carrying their babies by two hours per day.

One thing that does seem to reduce crying is introducing a flexible routine to a baby's waking hours, similar to the kind of approach suggested by "Baby Whisperer" Tracy Hogg. One study found that a repeated pattern in which naps were followed by a feed, then some interactive playtime, then some quiet time alone on a mat or in a playpen during which parents watched for any signs of tiredness (such as eye-rubbing) and put the baby back down for a sleep (either swaddled or tucked in tightly with sheets and blankets) reduced crying in babies under eight weeks of age.

Other studies have suggested that swaddling (or wrapping) the upper half of the body to restrict a baby's arm movements also seems to increase the amount of daytime sleep, although swaddled babies should never be placed facedown, and the swaddling shouldn't be so tight that babies can't move their limbs. Skin-to-skin contact can reduce crying in very young infants, and there is some evidence that massage can reduce crying and boost sleep and relaxation in babies under six months of age.

If you've tried everything, can find nothing wrong, and your baby still won't stop crying, most pediatricians agree that you should put your child down somewhere safe and take a break. Sadly, a minority of babies seem prone to crying for no apparent reason. The good news is that most babies who cry a lot at five to six weeks are no more likely than quieter babies to continue being unsettled by the age of three months. Many will start sleeping through the night at this age.

. 91 .
Why do some belly buttons become "outies"?

Belly buttons are the shriveled-up remnant of the umbilical cord, but just why some of them end up sticking out when others form a deep hole remains something of a mystery. One theory is that the "outieness" is influenced by the amount of scar tissue that forms underneath and around the severed umbilical cord. "Outies" can form because the opening to the cord doesn't close up properly, resulting in something called an umbilical hernia. Such hernias are usually painless, are more visible when a baby is crying or has a particularly full belly, and often disappear by about eighteen months of age.

There's currently no way of predicting whether your baby will have an outie. Around 20 percent of newborns have them, but many will turn into innies as the babies age and fat accumulates around the stalk of the scar, pulling it inward. Malnutrition can change the shape of the hood on top of the navel, while the size of the belly button is thought to relate to the size of the umbilical cord during pregnancy and may therefore signal how many nutrients the fetus received

Aki Sinkkonen of the University of Helsinki in Finland has researched the evolution of belly buttons and believes they may provide a signal about a woman's reproductive fitness (apparently, no one has done an equivalent study of male belly buttons). Studies suggest that the most desirable shape for a female belly button is a symmetrical "T" or vertical shape, with a large hood of skin at the top and neither excessively big nor small. However, Sinkkonen says that outies are common and socially appreciated in sub-Saharan Africa.

. 92 .
Do babies heal faster than adults?

Injuries are a fact of life, but the first time you spot blood oozing from your baby's perfect peachy skin is a traumatic event for any parent, especially if the injury is your own fault. The first time it happened to me, I was trimming my month-old daughter's fingernails and accidentally nipped the skin, which produced an obscene amount of blood for such a trivial injury.

The miraculous thing is that babies seem to heal with little or no scarring. Injure an adult's skin, and the body releases chemicals that promote swelling and inflammation, rallying immune cells to the scene. As the skin begins to heal, cells secrete collagen fibers to patch up the wound; whereas in normal skin, these collagen fibers form a crisscross pattern, in scar tissue, they are laid down in parallel bundles, making the tissue less flexible. In contrast, the immune system of the fetus is immature, and there is very little inflammation when the skin is injured, which seems to allow it to heal better. Even when relatively major operations are performed on fetuses in the uterus, they can be born blemish-free.

This superior healing ability seems to extend beyond birth. In a recent study, doctors at the Children's Hospital of Philadelphia analyzed samples of human foreskin removed during circumcision. They were curious to know why it is that the amount of scarring and the number of complications they see following routine operations to repair hypospadias—a common birth defect in which the hole at the end of the penis is in the wrong place—increase as children age.

When they analyzed skin from babies younger than twenty-eight days old, they found that it produced far lower levels of chemicals known to promote inflammation than skin from six- to twelve-month-olds. The amounts of these chemicals were even higher in older children.

It's not just scarring. Recent studies have shown that if the tip of a newborn mouse's heart is surgically removed, within a matter of weeks, it will have grown back. Further investigation revealed that the remaining heart cells started to divide and create new muscle tissue—something that would be unthinkable in adults. Although no one has proved yet that human babies have the same abilities, pediatric surgeons report that certain types of heart surgery are far more successful when performed within the first few months of birth than if they wait until the baby is older. If we can understand the complicated chemical signals that enable this regeneration to take place, we might one day be able to help adults achieve a similar feat.

. 93 .

Why do babies gnaw on things even before they start teething?

Red cheeks? Drooling and irritable? Chewing on anything they can get their hands on? The baby has to be teething, right? Many other symptoms are attributed to teething, including diarrhea, sleep disturbances, and fever. But is teething really the villain it's made out to be?

Babies are actually born with their milk teeth already sitting in a neat row beneath the gum, but most babies don't cut their first teeth until about six months of age (in rare cases, babies are born with visible teeth, much to the dismay of moms who had intended to breast-feed). First to appear are the central (cutting) incisors, followed soon afterward by the lateral incisors that sit next to them, then the first molars and the canines. At around the age of two, the second set of molars starts to appear. Girls tend to get their teeth earlier than boys, although the reason for this is unknown.

Just what causes teeth to erupt from the gum remains a medical mystery, but we do know that teeth aren't pushed upward by the growth of the root or the jawbone. The tooth itself seems to be a passive bystander in the process, but the structure from which it emerges in the jaw is capable of producing all sorts of chemicals that can prompt cell growth and inflammation, and these could theoretically trigger the irritation, drooling, and vivid red cheeks considered a sign of teething. Indeed, some of these chemicals have been linked to fever and to disturbances in sleep and appetite.

Though several studies have suggested that babies who are teething show more mouthing, sucking, drooling, and fever than nonteething babies, these studies suffer from the fact that the people making the observations knew they were participating in a study about teething and therefore may have been biased.

To investigate further, Melissa Wake and her colleagues at the Royal Children's Hospital in Parkville, Australia, asked the parents of twenty-one babies attending day-care centers to fill out daily questionnaires describing their child's mood, wellness, drooling, sleep, the contents of their diapers, and any rashes or facial flushing they'd noticed over the previous twenty-four hours. The parents and nursery staff dutifully completed these questionnaires for seven months, and every day a dental therapist came to take the babies' temperature and check them for any signs of tooth eruption.

Contrary to widespread belief, the researchers found no evidence for increased illness or fever, mood or sleep disturbances, drooling, strong urine, red cheeks, or rashes in the five days leading up to the eruption of a tooth and on the day itself—although parents did report looser stools in the five days leading up to the appearance of a tooth.

More recently, Brazilian researchers conducted a similar study of forty-seven babies being cared for by their mothers at home. They found some

evidence of increased sleep disturbance, drooling, rash, runny nose, diarrhea, loss of appetite, and irritability on the day of tooth eruption and one
day afterward. However, these symptoms weren't present in the days running
up to it, meaning there was no way of predicting when teeth might put in an
appearance.

So why are these findings so different from what we have been led to believe? Wake says that teething may have become a scapegoat for many other
events occurring between the ages of six and twenty-four months, including
a sudden rise in respiratory, middle-ear, and diarrheal infections, as well as
other developmental processes that could cause babies to be more irritable
than normal or to sleep less.

If a baby is being fussy and irritable, it can be easier to attribute it to a
known physical cause than to accept that she's simply in a bad mood—or
that there is a behavioral problem that should be addressed. I know my own
daughter has generated far more sympathy from me if she has been whiny
and difficult and sporting red cheeks, compared to when there is no obvious
physical cause.

. 94 .
Why is baby hair a different color from adult hair,
and why do babies lose their hair?

Some babies are born bald, while others are born sporting a full head of hair
that may bear no relation to the color it will be a few months later (let alone
when the child becomes an adult). My daughter, Matilda, was born semi-
bald but with a fringe of brown hair around the base of her scalp that made
her look a bit like a monk. A month later, this fell out and was replaced with a
mop of silky blond hair. A friend's daughter was born with bright-orange hair;
she, too, is now blond.

A baby's hair begins to grow from around twenty weeks of pregnancy, and
the first hair they produce—vellus hair—tends to be silky and fine and similar to the hair that grows on the rest of our bodies. As the hair follicles on the
head grow larger, this early hair begins to be replaced with intermediate hair,

although some of the early baby hair continues to grow. At around the age of two, intermediate hair is replaced by thicker terminal hair that is more similar in texture to adult hair.

A pigment called melanin plays a large role in determining hair color, and there are two types: eumelanin, which colors hair brown to black; and pheomelanin, which colors hair blond to red. In general, your hair color depends on the proportion of these pigments that your body possesses. Many blond children end up with darker hair as adults. This is because the enzyme that makes these pigments becomes more active as people age, and under the influence of hormones that start being produced at puberty.

Although no one has tested this, it could well be that the hormones coursing through Mom's body during pregnancy mean that a baby's first hair is a different color from the later hair. We know that high levels of estrogen from the mother's body sometimes cause baby girls to have swollen breasts and even produce milk or menstruate during the first days after birth.

So what causes some babies to lose their hair? Hair usually starts growing at the front of the head and spreads backward as the baby gets older. It also runs in cycles, consisting of a growing phase, an intermediate phase, and a resting phase, after which the hair falls out. How much hair a baby is born with depends on what stage of this cycle their hair follicles have reached. Some babies will have lost all their vellus hair by the time they are born (and started growing new hair), while others will be left with a bit of vellus hair—usually toward the back of the head, like Matilda was born with.

These growth cycles can overlap to some degree, which means that babies can have a mixture of different hair types at the same time. As a general rule, babies with darker skin tend to have longer cycles of hair growth, so they are often born with fuller heads of hair than fair babies.

One patch of hair toward the back of the scalp has a stubborn tendency not to enter its final resting phase until around three months after birth. Many parents notice a bald patch of skin on the back of their baby's head around this time, which is usually blamed on babies rubbing their heads against their crib mattresses. Although rubbing the area probably helps the hair to fall out, this bald patch is actually caused by the shedding of this final patch of vellus hair. The phenomenon has a catchy name: occipital neonatal alopecia.

. 95 .
Can newborns sweat?

Babies are capable of regulating their internal body temperature from birth (unless they're very premature), although they're not as good at it as adults. One of the mechanisms they use is sweating, which causes heat to be lost by evaporation. Studies have shown that most babies born after thirty-six weeks are capable of sweating from day one, although they don't sweat as much as adults and may need higher temperatures to trigger it. This means that sweating isn't a good guide to how hot a baby is, and you're better off feeling the back of the neck or chest to get an indication of temperature.

. 96 .
Do fontanelles hurt?

The skull is made up of seven bones, but these aren't joined up at birth. This means a baby's head can change shape and be slightly compressed as it makes its way through the birth canal, making it easier for the baby to be born. The areas where these bones join are called the fontanelles (or soft spots), although there are only really two that are big enough for you to feel. The most obvious one is located on the top of the head, feels like a soft diamond, and will remain there for up to nineteen months, although you may feel another small one at the back of the head that usually closes after two months. As well as enabling the head to be compressed, the fontanelles allow the brain some room to grow, before the bones of the skull eventually join up and harden.

It's difficult to know how hard you'd have to press the fontanelles for it to hurt your baby (and I doubt many would want to try). Although clearly not as solid as bone, they're relatively robust, as the brain is protected by a thick fibrous membrane that stands between it and the skin.

. 97 .
Are pacifiers good or bad for babies?

The fashion for pacifiers waxes and wanes. Right now in middle-class Britain, there seems to be a look of disapproval for any baby spotted with a pacifier in its mouth, even though many a grandmother swears by them to soothe crying babies and settle them to sleep. Even so, an estimated 75 to 85 percent of babies in Western countries use a pacifier, at least in private.

So who is right? There's no doubt that young babies love to suck (be it on a thumb or on a piece of molded plastic), and pediatricians widely regard sucking as one of the best ways of relieving pain in young babies.

The evidence for pacifiers helping to ward off sudden infant death syndrome (SIDS) is pretty compelling—to the extent that the American Academy of Pediatrics now recommends offering a pacifier at naptime and bedtime to reduce the risk of SIDS. Studies have estimated that one SIDS death could be prevented for every 2,733 babies who use a pacifier when put down to sleep. There are several theories as to why this might be. One is that babies sleeping with a pacifier seem to be easier to arouse, so they might be more likely to wake up if something happens to them during the night. Another theory is that a pacifier makes it easier for a baby to breathe through its mouth if its nose becomes blocked. However, pediatricians do not recommend forcing a baby to use a pacifier if it doesn't want to, or reinserting it if the baby spits it out.

The risk of SIDS is greatest in babies up to the age of six months, so after this, the health benefits of using a pacifier start to fade. One reason to wean babies off them is a slightly increased risk of other infections. Several studies have found that pacifiers are often colonized with yeast and bacteria, and latex pacifiers seem to allow more of these organisms to flourish than silicone ones. Sucking a thumb or fingers can increase a baby's exposure to such organisms, although no one has directly compared whether this is any better or worse than pacifier-sucking.

While most of these organisms won't cause disease, a study of more than ten thousand babies in the UK found that those who sucked either a pacifier or their fingers at the age of fifteen months had a higher incidence of earache and colic compared with those who didn't—although it's possible that pacifiers were being used to calm babies who got sick for different reasons. The effect is likely to be small, though. Another study of 476 children found that 35 percent of those who used pacifiers developed at least one middle-ear infection, compared to 32 percent of those who didn't suck, while rates of recurrent ear infection were 16 percent in the pacifier group, compared to 11 percent among controls.

Finally, many parents worry about the effect that pacifiers or thumb-sucking might be having on their child's mouth development. Both the American Dental Association and the American Academy of Pediatric Dentistry recommend that pacifiers be discouraged after four years of age because of an increased risk of malocclusion, or misalignment of the teeth. In one study, the prevalence of malocclusion was around 71 percent in children who used a pacifier or sucked their thumb for more than four years, compared with 32 percent in children who stopped sucking between the age of three and four, and just 14 percent in those who stopped sucking before the age of two.

Sleep

. 98 .
Can babies tell the difference between night and day?

Newborns tend to sleep a lot—at least for the first couple of weeks, which comes as a relief to their shell-shocked parents. The average newborn crams in around sixteen to eighteen hours of sleep per day, which tends to drop to around fourteen to fifteen hours by the time they are a month old. At this stage, a newborn's sleep patterns are more influenced by the fullness of its belly than by whether it's light or dark outside, but by two or three months, it is beginning to grasp the notion of night and day.

As anyone who has suffered from jet lag will know, we humans have a firmly entrenched body clock, which means our bodies respond differently depending on what time of day it is. As night falls, we produce more of the sleep-promoting hormone melatonin, which makes us increasingly drowsy as the evening progresses.

So what about babies? The body's master clock is located at the front of the brain in an area called the suprechiasmic nucleus (SCN). It is in direct contact with the eyes and can be shifted forward or backward by exposure to bright light, which is how the body manages to reset itself within a couple of days when you travel across time zones. The SCN is thought to have developed by around twenty weeks of pregnancy, and fetuses do show differences in their heart rates, breathing movements, and hormone levels depending on the time of day—although these rhythms are probably being driven by signals from the mother, rather than being self-generated.

The SCN continues gradually to mature after birth. For the first few weeks, a baby's sleep is distributed pretty evenly over twenty-four hours, but by six weeks, most babies are slightly more active during the day and sleepier at night, and by three months, higher levels of melatonin can be detected in a baby's blood at night.

Your grandmother may tell you that a good way of getting a baby to sleep through the night is to stick it outside in the garden during the daytime. Although you may be suspicious that this is simply a ruse for the mother to get some peace and quiet, Grandma might be correct: Research has shown that two- to three- month-olds who are exposed to plenty of bright sunlight during the day sleep better at night. This is probably for the same reason that people overcome jet lag faster if they get outdoors into the sunshine—bright light plays a crucial role in setting the body's central clock and ensuring that it runs on time.

. 99 .
Are a baby's sleep patterns inherited?

Most people broadly fall into one of two categories: early birds, who wake up early and like to turn in to bed soon after it gets dark; and night owls, who like to slumber through the morning and are more active during the evening. Just which category you fall into seems to be inherited, to some degree, which is good news for owl-like parents who dread being woken up by a "dawn baby chorus."

Interestingly, just how much of an early bird or night owl someone becomes also seems to be driven by the season in which they were born. Several European and Canadian studies have suggested that babies born during spring and summer are more likely to turn into night owls, while those born in autumn and winter are more likely to become early birds. The effect was particularly strong among babies born in Montreal during late September and October, a high proportion of whom became morning types. This might be explained by the fact that the months from October to December tend to be gloomy for those living in Montreal, with the lowest average hours of sunshine over the year. Researchers believe that there may be a critical window of time after birth when the body clock is extremely sensitive to light and its future pattern can be set. Studies in rats have suggested that those raised in dim light are more sensitive to its effects, finding it harder to sleep during daylight, for example.

What about other aspects of sleep? Much of what we know about the inheritance of sleep patterns comes from studies of identical twins. Because they share the same genes, you can look at differences in twins' behavior to calculate what proportion comes down to genetics and what proportion can be attributed to external factors such as how they were raised, the hours they work, and their social lives. Twin studies have suggested that approximately a third of the difference in the amount of sleep people need, the amount of time it takes people to fall asleep, and how often they wake during the night can be explained by genetic factors. This means that although a baby's sleep patterns should show some relation to how you sleep as parents, external factors have a greater influence.

. 100 .
How can I get my baby to sleep through the night?

The average newborn sleeps sixteen to eighteen hours a day, but there is a lot of variability among individuals. One large study found that some newborns slept for just nine hours per day, while others clocked up a whopping nineteen hours of sleep over twenty-four hours. The same is true at two months of age, with some babies sleeping for just twelve hours a day and others managing twenty-one.

The good news for parents who find themselves blessed with a sleepy newborn is that the amount of sleep babies need and their general degree of fussiness seems to remain relatively consistent as they get older—although how often they wake, feed, and cry can vary according to what's going on in their lives.

As for sleeping through the night, parents shouldn't expect too much too soon. Though studies have found that up to three quarters of babies are sleeping through the night by twelve weeks of age, what "sleeping through the night" means to researchers is five hours of undisturbed sleep in a row—a definition I suspect most parents would find reason to quibble with. A review of twenty-six studies focusing on babies' sleep found that just 37 percent of healthy three-month-olds regularly slept for eight hours at night without waking their parents.

While the amount of sleep a baby needs is inherited, to some degree, research suggests that parents' interactions with the baby play a crucial role in terms of getting it to sleep through the night. So how do you encourage your baby to fall into the sleepy category?

Most sleep researchers agree that introducing a consistent bedtime routine in the run-up to bed, such as brushing teeth, taking a bath, and reading a story, helps babies to fall asleep, as do waking them at the same time each morning (assuming they don't wake you first) and ensuring that they get some kind of physical exercise during the day. Making a clear distinction between night- and daytime seems to help, for example, by settling babies for naps in rooms that aren't too dark during the daytime and minimizing interaction at night. At least one study found that babies exposed to more natural light in the early afternoon slept better at night than those exposed to less.

Babies are creatures of habit and quickly learn to associate certain cues with sleep. This means that if parents aren't careful, they can form bad habits. A review of studies on night waking and other bedtime issues found that some of the most common problems included needing to be rocked or held or for the parent to be present in order for the baby to fall asleep; needing to be fed to sleep; and habitually waking several times during the night. It is unlikely that parents set out to form such habits; more likely, they are born out of desperation—taking a baby into bed and breast-feeding it back to sleep when it wakes for the fifth hour in a row, for example.

Trying to prevent bad habits from forming in the first place can be easier than trying to break them once they've become established. Most experts agree that parents should try to put a baby down in its crib while still awake so the baby doesn't become reliant on their presence in order to fall asleep.

There are a few other tactics that parents can use to try to establish good sleep habits from a tender age. A study of 610 women found that those who were taught the following techniques when their babies were ten days old were 10 percent more likely to have a baby who slept consistently for five hours or more at twelve weeks, compared to parents who received little or no advice.

(The next eight points are taken from "Use of a behavioral programme in the first three months to prevent infant crying and sleeping problems," *Journal of Paediatrics and Child Health,* June 2001, vol. 37, issue 3, pp. 289–97.)

1. During the daytime, feed your baby whenever she seems hungry, and spend plenty of time interacting with her. Try to bathe her at around the same time each day.

2. Encourage your baby to take a "focal feed"—either a longer than normal breast-feed or a larger formula feed—between ten P.M. and midnight.

3. If your baby is still awake after feeding and changing, try not to hold, rock, or nurse him to sleep. Instead, put him into the crib while he's still awake and leave him to settle himself. Lights should be dimmed, although it doesn't have to be completely dark.

4. If your baby doesn't settle, check the following:
   (a) Does the diaper need changing?
   (b) Does he need to be burped?
   (c) Is he too hot or cold?
   (d) Stroke and talk softly to your baby. If necessary, pick him up and have a cuddle.

Give each tactic at least ten minutes to work before moving on to the next one.

5. Try to distinguish between genuine crying and fretting in order to reduce the number of times your baby is picked up at night. Babies may fret before settling to sleep and don't always need further attention.

6. Try to keep the lights dimmed during night feeds. Respond to your baby's needs by changing the diaper or feeding her and then settle her back to bed. If your baby doesn't settle, work through step 4 again. Avoid playing or socializing with your baby.
7. If your baby is waking more than every three to four hours at night, he probably don't need the diaper changed every time.
8. Make nights as uninteresting as possible for your baby. Nighttime is for sleeping.

Once babies were three weeks old (so long as they were healthy and gaining weight), moms were told to start lengthening the time between night feeds. This didn't mean leaving babies to "cry it out" for long periods on their own, but teaching them to dissociate waking and feeding so they didn't automatically expect to be fed if they woke at night. Delaying tactics included changing the diaper, resettling them back to sleep, patting, or carrying them. (Note: The current advice from breast-feeding experts is to resist cutting out night feeds for at least the first few weeks of breast-feeding, when feeding on demand is necessary to establish a good and regular supply of milk.)

Many of the women in this study didn't bother with the prolonged evening feed, presumably because they felt uneasy about waking a baby who was already asleep. They also took closer to six weeks to start lengthening the space between night feeds. Still, the fact that there was a difference between the groups suggests there are measures that parents can take to boost nighttime sleep.

The use of focal feeds (also known as "dream feeds") was investigated in a separate (although small) study of twenty-six women and their newborn babies, half of whom were told to give an extra-large feed between ten P.M. and midnight and then to gradually increase the amount of time between night feeds by resettling the baby without feeding if it woke at night by swaddling or changing the diaper. The mothers also tried to settle babies in the crib for daytime naps rather than carrying them and tried to maximize differences between night and daytime (for example, by not using blackout blinds during the day and trying to engage as little as possible at night).

By the time these babies reached eight weeks, all of those following the program were sleeping for regular five-hour stretches at night, compared to just 23 percent of babies who weren't. Even though the babies were feeding less frequently at night, the researchers found that their weight gain and overall milk intake over twenty-four hours was the same as for babies who fed more often. They seemed to make up for the reduced night feeds by drinking more milk in the early morning.

. 101 .
Is co-sleeping good or bad for my baby?

Co-sleeping is the norm for around 90 percent of the world's population, yet child-care experts in many Western countries advise against it. Part of the reason is safety, since studies have linked co-sleeping to a slightly increased risk of sudden infant death syndrome (SIDS), although steps can be taken to reduce the risk. However, there's also a prevailing fear that if babies start off sleeping in the parental bed, it will become impossible to kick them out of it.

Despite these fears, co-sleeping seems to be on the increase in many Western countries. One survey of U.S. parents found that the number of mothers co-sleeping with their baby for all or part of the night doubled between 1993 and 2000 to 12.8 percent, while a separate study reported that nearly half of UK mothers share a bed with their baby at some point during the first month of its life; this drops to 29 percent when babies are three months old.

Those who champion co-sleeping claim that it makes breast-feeding easier, boosts the baby's development, and promotes bonding—and that it actually reduces the risk of SIDS, because parents can keep a closer eye on their baby. It is true that studies have found a higher rate of breast-feeding among mothers who share a bed with their baby compared to babies who sleep alone, although it's difficult to disentangle the fact that many women who choose to co-sleep are also keen to breast-feed. One small study that filmed babies either sharing a bed with their moms, lying in an open-sided crib that was attached to the bed, or lying in a separate cot found that those in the bed or crib attempted to feed more often and had more successful feeds than those in the separate cot, which could help establish a better milk supply. However, a separate study found no difference in the rate at which babies gained weight between co-sleepers and babies who slept in cribs.

Evidence that co-sleeping benefits brain development is also patchy. One study that followed 205 children from birth through to the age of eighteen found better cognitive performance in areas such as memory and decision-making among those who co-slept as babies when they reached the age of six, but the effect was small, and there was no difference in their cognitive, social, emotional or developmental maturity when they were assessed again at age eighteen. Meanwhile, a separate study of 175 babies who slept alone and 29 babies who routinely co-slept found that the solitary sleepers were generally less irritable than the co-sleepers when they were assessed at four months of age.

A key problem is that the definition of co-sleeping varies among researchers, health professionals, and parents. Researchers tend to define co-sleeping as sharing the same room rather than the same bed, while health professionals use co-sleeping to describe bed-sharing. Those who champion co-sleeping often cite a study that found higher self-esteem among women who co-slept as young children, but it actually looked at women who spent several years sleeping in their parents' bedroom, not necessarily sharing a bed with them. The fact is that very little good-quality research has been done on the physical or emotional benefits of co-sleeping, so the jury is out.

The issue of safety is also far from straightforward. Those studies that have looked at the characteristics of babies who died from SIDS have identified co-sleeping as a possible contributing factor, but it is difficult to disentangle it from other factors that go alongside bed-sharing, such as poverty, parents who smoke, or the baby sleeping on its front. Depending on the characteristics of individual families, estimates on the risk of SIDS for babies who share a bed with their parents ranges from no increased risk among nonsmoking families to a twelve-fold increased risk for babies sleeping on a sofa with a parent who smokes.

Given this uncertainty, it probably comes down to individual parents to decide what works best for them. If you do want to share a bed with your baby, factors that seem to increase the risk of SIDS include smoking (particularly if the mother smoked during pregnancy, which may affect the development of the brain), sleeping with the baby on a sofa, and consuming drugs or alcohol. Overheating and smothering with pillows are possible risks, so take steps to prevent these from happening.

. 102 .
Will leaving my baby to cry cause any long-term damage?

No subject is more divisive among parents than controlled crying. Those who support it claim the pain is only temporary and that teaching babies to settle themselves is one of the greatest gifts a parent can give. Those who oppose it believe that leaving a child to cry is tantamount to cruelty and may cause lasting damage. Parenting books also disagree on the matter. Out of thirty-nine books on infant sleep that are currently available in the U.S., twenty-four endorse or advocate controlled crying as a means of teaching children to sleep, while twelve oppose or warn against it. The remainder take no position.

In terms of teaching babies to sleep, controlled crying does seem to work, although other, less severe methods appear to be equally effective. In 2006, the American Academy of Sleep Medicine (AASM) published a review of fifty-two studies that evaluated the effectiveness of various methods of sleep training, many of which involved some degree of controlled crying.

In its strictest form, controlled crying (also known as "extinction" or "crying it out") involves ignoring all crying, tantrums, and calls for parents, unless the child is hurt, ill, or in danger—and doing this every night, no matter how long the crying lasts. The claim is that if you cave in and respond to the child, it will simply learn to cry longer the next time. Softer variations include leaving progressively longer intervals before going in and reassuring the child, then leaving; or staying in the room with the child but ignoring its cries. The ultimate goal is to teach the child to develop its own self-soothing skills so it can fall asleep independently of its parents.

Other strategies for teaching children to sleep involve establishing positive bedtime routines, such as taking a bath and reading a story; scheduled awakenings, when a child is deliberately roused fifteen to thirty minutes before it would usually wake up, then settled back down while semi-conscious; and educating parents about establishing regular naptimes, consistent bedtime routines, and putting babies into their cribs when they're drowsy but not asleep.

According to the AASM review, all of these strategies worked to some degree, and of the few studies that conducted head-to-head comparisons of the different methods, there was little evidence to suggest that any were vastly superior in terms of effectiveness in the long run. Strict controlled crying seemed to work faster than scheduled awakenings in babies who woke often at night, but the different forms of controlled crying seemed to be pretty much on a level playing field in terms of teaching babies to sleep, along with establishing positive bedtime routines.

Parents should consider a baby's age before considering any form of sleep training.

Babies younger than three months

At least two randomized controlled trials have found that trying to use any form of sleep training on babies younger than three months is ineffective and doesn't decrease crying. There are steps you can take to prevent bad habits from forming (see 100: "How can I get my baby to sleep through the night?").

Babies three to six months

Most experts agree that controlled crying shouldn't be used on babies under six months of age, as they may need to feed during the night. You might try working on establishing positive bedtime routines and making sure your baby gets regular naps during the day—or try scheduled awakenings if your baby wakes often during the night.

Babies older than six months

If you and your baby still aren't getting enough sleep and you're considering controlled crying, you can take comfort from several studies that have investigated whether it has any long-term adverse effects. The general conclusion is that, overall, sleep training makes babies more secure, more predictable, and less irritable than they were before treatment. An Australian study of 225 babies whose parents used controlled crying at eight to ten months of age found that controlled crying reduced babies' sleep problems by around 30 percent within four months, although 15 percent of babies didn't respond to it. When parents completed questionnaires assessing their children's emotional and behavioral development at various points until the age of six, there seemed to be no difference between children who had received sleep training as infants and those who hadn't.

There is one final note of caution. In 2012, a study was published suggesting that controlled crying did have a short-term physical effect on a baby's stress levels even after it had stopped crying out for its parents at night. Wendy Middlemiss and her colleagues at the University of North Texas measured daily levels of the stress hormone cortisol in twenty-four babies aged four to ten months as they underwent a five-day residential sleep-training program at a hospital in New Zealand. The program involved a typical regime of controlled crying in which mother and baby were separated at bedtime and a nurse settled the baby into its crib. It was then left to fall asleep by itself, although a nurse would go in and check on the baby every ten minutes if it continued to cry. The mother was not allowed to comfort the baby but was in a nearby room and could hear its cries.

Levels of cortisol were similar in moms and babies before sleep training commenced; perhaps unsurprisingly, they rose considerably after the first night. The same thing happened on the second night, but by the third night, the babies had learned to settle themselves to sleep and cried considerably less. At this point, the mothers' cortisol levels began to fall, and they expressed relief that their babies were beginning to respond to sleep training and they were finally getting a decent night's sleep. However, measurements of cortisol revealed a disconnection between the babies' outwardly calm appearance and what was going on inside. Although the babies no longer cried, they continued to experience high levels of cortisol, similar to those on the first night. This might suggest that, though they're calm on the outside, they are unhappy on the inside.

No further measures of cortisol were taken after the program ended, so it's impossible to know at this stage whether the babies' stress levels eventually normalized—although the fact that other studies have found no lasting negative effects from controlled crying is somewhat reassuring. Further studies are clearly needed to confirm how long babies remain stressed. "It may well be that the infant is still in a transition period and will be fine," says Middlemiss, "but the disturbing thing for me is that the mother can't choose whether or not to respond to the infant's distress, because she can't see it."

Given that less severe forms of controlled crying seem to be just as effective as the strict version in terms of curbing sleep problems, I'd personally be tempted to try one of these variations first.

. 103 .
What's more effective: introducing strict routines or immediately responding to my baby's demands?

As with controlled crying, parents tend to split over whether babies should adhere to strict schedules or have Mom and Dad at their beck and call. In *The New Contented Little Baby Book,* Gina Ford suggests that in order to get your baby to sleep through the night from an early age, you need to establish the right associations and structure your baby's feeds and naps from the day you arrive home from the hospital. At the opposite end of the spectrum, attachment-parenting gurus such as Jean Liedloff advocate prolonged holding, frequent breast-feeding, co-sleeping, and rapidly responding to a baby's cries in order to foster strong emotional bonds between mother and baby.

In a recent study, Ian St. James-Roberts and colleagues at the Thomas Coram Research Unit in London compared the impact of these very different parenting styles on the amount of time young babies spent crying and sleeping. They recruited three groups of parents: one from London, one from Copenhagen, and a third group of mixed-nationality parents who practiced an extreme form of attachment parenting (also known as proximal care), in which babies were carried around for much of the day, breast-fed on demand, and parents rapidly responded to cries. Parents were asked to keep daily diaries of what they did and how their babies responded at various points during the baby's first twelve weeks. They also completed questionnaires about infant feeding and sleeping patterns. Parents in the proximal-care group spent around sixteen and a half hours a day holding their ten-day-old babies and fed them fourteen times a day, while London parents tended toward the tough-love approach, holding babies around half this amount of time and spacing out feeds so they ate eleven times a day. Babies in Copenhagen fell somewhere in between, held for nearly ten hours a day and fed twelve times. London parents also left their baby to cry for around three times longer each day than either the Copenhagen or proximal-care parents.

At twelve weeks of age, 85 percent of proximal-care and 70 percent of Copenhagen babies were still exclusively breast-fed, compared to just 37 percent of London babies (though this could be for cultural reasons), and most proximal-care parents co-slept with their infants, while just 16 percent of Copenhagen parents and 9 percent of London parents did the same.

So how did the babies respond? Those living in London spent around 50 percent more time fussing and crying than those in the other groups, though there was no difference in bouts of inconsolable crying (see 89: "What causes colic?"). When parents were asked how many nights in the past week their twelve-week-old baby had slept for five hours or more, London and Copenhagen parents reported around five such nights, while proximal-care parents reported just three and a half nights on average.

This is just one study, but it does suggest that the extreme form of proximal care is more likely to result in frazzled parents, without any obvious benefit in terms of sleep quality or the amount of time babies spend crying, compared to the more moderate approach of the Danes. By the parents quickly responding to their baby's cries, the Danish babies spent less time crying overall (although we don't know if extra crying is actually harmful to babies), and they seemed to sleep just as well. On the other hand, the tough-love approach of the London parents didn't mean they got any less sleep—they just may have had to put up with sore eardrums during the day.

The White Stuff

. 104 .
How does breast-feeding work?

It's one of the most natural processes in the world, yet until very recently, the mechanism by which babies manage to extract milk from the breast was unclear. Some thought babies squeezed milk out of the nipples by kneading them in their mouths—much as a milkmaid squeezes milk from a cow's udder—while others proposed that the milk was removed by suction.

In 2010, Australian researchers finally solved the mystery after combining ultrasound imaging of babies suckling on the breast with measurements of the vacuum created by their mouths. "It's not a milking action at all," says Donna Geddes of the University of Western Australia in Crawley, who led the research. "What we see is that when the tongue is lowered and the vacuum is applied, that's when the milk is coming out of the breast."

They found that babies who struggle to breast-feed generate far weaker vacuums than those who breast-feed successfully, which may help explain why premature babies often struggle to feed: Their mouth muscles aren't strong enough yet to create a vacuum. The study emphasizes the point that painful crushing or distortion of the nipple isn't necessary for breast-feeding to occur. If your nipples are coming out of your baby's mouth distorted, this probably means that your baby isn't latching on correctly, and you should try repositioning them or speak to a lactation consultant.

. 105 .
Should I feed on demand or wait three to four hours between feeds?

It's pretty much undisputed that if you plan to breast-feed, you should try to feed whenever your baby appears hungry, for at least the first couple of weeks. The amount of milk that women produce six days after birth is strongly linked to the volume they will produce at six weeks, so it seems that frequent stimulation of the breasts during these very early days is needed to get the breasts producing enough milk. If you start substituting breast feeds with formula milk, then your milk production will start to fall.

But what about once breast-feeding has been successfully established? Women are usually told to "feed on demand" without being told what this means. Does it mean feed whenever the baby cries? Or only when the baby is hungry, in which case, how do you know if the baby is hungry rather than tired or uncomfortable? There is no hard-and-fast rule. Studies have shown that individual babies show a three-fold variation in the amount of milk they consume per day, as well as a wide variation in their patterns of milk intake. By the age of one month, the average baby drinks 750 to 800 milliliters of milk per day, but a recent Australian study found that, although babies under six months fed eight times every twenty-four hours on average, some took as few as four feeds and others as many as thirteen feeds during this time.

Having gotten the hang of breast-feeding, many women want to try to space out feeds, particularly at night. When this study compared the amount of breast milk consumed by babies who did and didn't feed during the night, it found no significant difference in the total amount of milk they consumed over twenty-four hours. The main difference was that the night feeders drank the biggest quantities of milk at night, while those who skipped night feeds drank more in the morning to compensate. This should serve to reassure women that if their baby doesn't feed during the night, it probably will be getting enough to eat overall.

Other common worries include whether babies who take frequent small breast feeds are getting enough high-fat milk to fill them up, and whether there is enough milk in the breasts to satisfy the appetite. Once breast-feeding is established, the average breast holds six ounces of milk, or almost twice the amount most babies will consume at a single sitting. However, the storage capacity of individual women ranges from 2.5 ounces to 13 ounces per breast. In general, women with bigger storage capacities give feeds less often, but not always. So you shouldn't assume that your baby is asking to feed more often because you're not making enough milk to quench its thirst. Nor does there seem to be much relationship between the size of your breasts before pregnancy—or how much the breasts grow during pregnancy—and how much milk they can store. Indeed, studies have found that the amount of breast growth during pregnancy is relatively consistent among mothers, regardless of their original breast size. "Of course, if the breasts are very small, they will not be able to store a large amount of milk, but apart from that, there will be no relationship between bra size and breast-milk storage capacity," says Jacqueline Kent of the University of Western Australia, who researches how breast-feeding works. One way of estimating how much milk your breasts contain is to use a breast pump to empty them before you would usually feed your baby, then give the milk to the baby in a bottle, although this is only a rough guide, as pumps don't extract as much milk as babies do—particularly if, like me, you find them uncomfortable to use for more than around ten minutes at a time, when your baby would feed for longer.

In general, the fat content of breast milk changes as babies progress through a feed, starting with more watery foremilk and progressing to richer hindmilk, but how much it changes varies according to how often women give feeds. Studies show that when babies take six to nine large feeds per day, the fat content changes from around 4.3 percent at the start of the feed to 10.7 percent by the end, but the foremilk tends to be richer in women who give feeds more frequently. When babies take fourteen to eighteen small feeds each day, the foremilk contains around 4.8 percent fat and the hindmilk around 8.2 percent fat. Regardless of how often they feed, there seems to be little difference in the total amount of fat that babies receive.

That said, some common breast-feeding advice—such as allowing the baby to feed for only ten minutes per breast and not allowing "comfort suckling," which usually occurs toward the end of a feed and can be felt as rapid flutter-like sucks and periodic swallows—may reduce a baby's chances of getting its fill of creamy hindmilk. If you're uncertain whether your baby has fully drained the first breast and should be offered the second, the best measure is whether or not you can still hear him swallowing, says Pamela Douglas, a breast-feeding expert at the University of Queensland in Australia. If he has stopped swallowing, that probably means he has finished feeding, but you should try offering the second breast to make sure.

. 106 .
Is breast really best for babies?

The mantra that breast is best probably is true, at least for the first few months of a baby's life. The most convincing evidence for the superiority of breast milk over formula relates to the prevention of stomach and respiratory infections, including colds, flu, and diarrhea, among breast-fed babies. This is especially important in developing countries, where it may be harder to sterilize bottles and find clean water to prepare formula, and where diarrhea or lung infections may quickly become life-threatening as a result of inadequate medical care. It was largely for these reasons that the World Health Organization recommended that women should breast-feed exclusively for six months before starting to introduce solid foods, ideally continuing to breast-feed their baby until the age of two.

Even in developed countries, it is estimated that 53 percent of hospitalizations for diarrhea among babies could be prevented each month if everyone breast-fed their babies exclusively. Breast-feeding has been shown to cut the risk of necrotizing enterocolitis (a serious gastrointestinal disease that mostly affects preterm babies) by around 55 percent. It reduces the risk of hospitalizations for pneumonia by around 72 percent. Meanwhile, there's pretty good evidence that breast-feeding cuts the risk of SIDS by around 36 percent—even though no one really understands what causes it.

Mild diarrhea aside, all of these illnesses are relatively rare in developed countries, so if you can't breast-feed, for whatever reason, it's unlikely that your baby will come to harm through drinking formula. For example, in the case of SIDS, it is estimated that fifty-five hundred children would have to be breast-fed to prevent one death. And in the case of pneumonia, twenty-six would have to be breast-fed for four or more months to prevent one hospitalization. Breast-feeding is no guarantee against illness—it merely reduces the risk—and the protection lasts only as long as the woman is breast-feeding and ends soon after she stops.

Of course, the majority of women stop breast-feeding long before the two years recommended by the WHO, often for practical reasons such as having to return to work. Though many women struggle to breast-feed in the first place, for most, it is with an extremely guilty heart that they resort to the bottle.

Are they right to feel guilty? Besides reducing the risk of infections in the short term, there are plenty of claims for additional benefits of breast-feeding. Many health organizations, including the American Academy of Pediatrics and the UK's National Health Service, state that breast-feeding also offers long-term protection against obesity, eczema, and diabetes. Others, such as the website Ask Dr. Sears, state that breast-feeding boosts IQ, eyesight, and response to vaccination, and reduces the risk of childhood cancer or the need for orthodontics.

However, once you start delving into the medical literature, it becomes clear that the evidence for breast being overwhelmingly better than bottle-feeding on these longer-term health measures is less clear-cut. For example, studies have shown that babies who are not breast-fed have 1.3 to 1.9 times as many allergy-related problems, are two to four times more likely to get (admittedly rare) childhood cancers, and are 1.2 to 1.6 times as likely to be overweight. A key problem is that many of these studies asked women to recall their breast-feeding habits from years ago, rather than monitoring children as they grow up, and their memories may have become clouded. When it comes to things like obesity, IQ, or high blood pressure, it is also difficult to disentangle socioeconomic factors, because mothers who breast-feed often come from different backgrounds than those who formula-feed.

The best way to take all of these factors into account would be to do a randomized controlled trial (RCT) in which similar women would be told either to breast-feed or formula-feed for a fixed period of time, and the health of their children would then be closely monitored for years afterward. No such trial has been done. For one thing, you can't tell women what to feed their babies. For another, many women who start off breast-feeding give up after a few weeks or months, or do complicated things such as breast-feeding during the daytime and introducing a bottle of formula at night.

Perhaps the closest anyone has come to this sort of RCT was a study of 16,491 women from Belarus conducted by Michael Kramer of McGill University in Montreal, Canada. In this study, half of the women were given advice and support regarding breast-feeding, while the remainder received no such help. This help worked to some extent—43 percent of women who received advice and support were breast-feeding exclusively when their babies were three months old, compared to just 6 percent in the control group. Like other research, it found that exclusive breast-feeding reduced the risk of gastrointestinal infection and eczema during infancy. However, when Kramer's team reexamined the children at six and a half, they found no difference in height or obesity, no reduction in blood pressure, allergy, asthma, or tooth decay, and no difference in behavior between the two groups.

These findings have since been backed up by a large study in the UK, which has been following the progress of more than 14,500 women and their babies since the early 1990s. Although it found that breast-feeding was associated with less obesity and lower blood pressure, it was impossible to separate this from the fact that women who breast-feed in the UK are more likely to come from middle- or upper-class backgrounds. When the same researchers looked at babies raised in Brazil, where breast-feeding isn't linked to social status, the links to obesity and blood pressure disappeared.

That's not to say that breast-feeding doesn't have long-term benefits; it's just that a lot more work needs to be done before we have a definitive answer. "In terms of a long-term effect on metabolism or the immune system, the evidence is either meager in terms of the number of studies, or conflicting because there are a lot of studies that don't agree," says Kramer. It's also likely that any protective effect will be small compared to more well-established risk factors, such as having a strong family history of obesity or disease.

However, there was one area where both Kramer and the Avon Longitudinal Study found strong evidence of a benefit: brain development. In Kramer's study, the breast-fed children scored around eight points higher on IQ tests when they were six and a half than those who were bottle-fed; unlike in many previous studies, the researchers had taken the mother's intelligence and socioeconomic background into account, so that couldn't explain the difference. "It's not really a delayed effect, because we know that the brain is largely developing in the uterus and during the first year or two of life," says Kramer. As for why breast-feeding should boost brain development, no one really knows. We don't even know if it's anything in the breast milk. "It could be a result of the physical contact between the mother and baby, or even increased verbal contact between the mother and baby during breast-feeding," Kramer says.

. 107 .
How long do I need to breast-feed in order for my baby to reap the benefits?

All moms want to do the best by their babies, but suggesting that they have to breast-feed for six months (let alone two years) or that they will be failing their children is not only unrealistic for most working mothers, it may not be supported by evidence regarding health benefits. "The strongest evidence for immediate breast-feeding benefits is exclusive breast-feeding for the first three to four months of life," says Ronald Kleinman, physician-in-chief at Massachusetts General Hospital for Children. "This impacts resistance to upper respiratory infections and diarrhea, and potentially improves responses to vaccines—although the evidence for this isn't as strong."

Studies that have found a reduction in the risk of SIDS followed babies for only six months, and the majority of SIDS deaths occur between the ages of two and four months.

As for longer-term benefits, such as protection against obesity or diabetes, the existing evidence also points to breast-feeding during the earliest months being key. For protection against allergic disease and type 1 diabetes, the mothers in the studies breast-fed for at least three to four months, while in the studies suggesting some degree of protection against childhood cancer, babies were breast-fed for six months.

After this, it's hard to know if additional breast-feeding offers significant long-term benefits for babies outside of the immediate protection it provides against infectious diseases, which, although important in developing countries, is arguably less of an issue in rich countries with adequate medical care. That's not to say that extended breast-feeding isn't beneficial, just that it has barely been studied—in part because so few women in Western countries do it. "There is really no solid evidence that introducing some formula at six months, or weaning from the breast and changing to formula at that time, has any health implications," Kleinman says.

One possible exception is brain development, where studies have indicated that babies get more benefit, the longer they are breast-fed. "At least in developing countries, there's evidence that breast-feeding beyond a year, or at least up to a year, is important," says Michael Kramer.

However, he emphasizes that women who don't breast-feed for this long should not necessarily feel guilty about it. "There are many other issues that are as important, if not probably more important, than breast-feeding," he says. For example, sitting your child in front of a TV and not playing with it is likely to have a bigger impact on its IQ than not breast-feeding. "In general, a happy mother is a better mother," says Kramer. "You're not guaranteed to be a good mother just because you follow the recommendations and breast-feed for two years."

Finally, women are often told that breast-feeding provides numerous benefits for their own health, such as protection against certain types of cancer, diabetes, or obesity (see 74: "Do women who breast-feed really lose their baby weight faster than those who bottle-feed?"). It's true that some studies have found health benefits, and the effect here seems to be cumulative—so it's the total amount of time you spend breast-feeding all of your babies that matters. For type 2 diabetes, there is a decreased risk of approximately 4 to 12 percent for every year of breast-feeding; while for breast and ovarian cancer, breast-feeding for longer than twelve months is associated with a 28 percent decrease in cancer risk.

. 108 .
Could combining breast- and formula-feeding offer babies the best of both worlds?

Whether it's the occasional bottle of formula if you're going out for the evening or a regular bottle to help your baby to sleep through the night, plenty of parents decide to combine breast-feeding with bottle-feeding. Some Latino communities even have a phrase for it: *los dos*. Many believe it offers the best of both worlds, combining the protective effects of breast-feeding with the additional nutrients of formula milk.

Despite its prevalence, such combination feeding has barely been studied. The World Health Organization doesn't distinguish it from the introduction of solid foods, despite the fact that the baby is getting all of its nutrients from milk. From their point of view, you either breast-feed exclusively or it doesn't count. But can you really have the best of both worlds? Those studies that have been done suggest that while combination feeding does provide some of the health benefits of breast-feeding, these are reduced. Take the common ear infection otitis media. Exclusive breast-feeding for longer than three months roughly halves the rate of ear infections, while in babies fed a combination of breast and formula milk, the risk is cut by around 23 percent. Exclusive breast-feeding also has roughly double the protective effect against sudden infant death syndrome (SIDS) compared to breast-feeding for some of the time. There's also some early evidence that breast milk produced in the evening may contain chemicals that help babies sleep, so if you do use formula for a nighttime "dream feed," you may miss out on this benefit (see 113: "Is morning breast milk any different from evening breast milk?").

What's not so clear is whether introducing the occasional bottle of formula milk makes it harder to maintain breast-feeding in the long term—a common concern of health professionals, because we know that frequent feeding in the early days is needed to establish a good milk supply. One study that compared babies fed a combination of breast and formula milk during the first week of life confirmed that the moms of combination-fed babies were less likely to continue breast-feeding, but only if they were white. Black and Hispanic mothers, on the other hand, seemed quite capable of continuing to combine breast- and bottle-feeding and were no less likely to have stopped breast-feeding by the time their babies reached three months of age.

This difference implies that the decision to switch from combination to formula-feeding is a cultural one, rather than the babies preferring the flavor of formula milk or refusing to take the breast after sucking on an artificial teat (see 110: "Does 'nipple confusion' really exist?"). In other words, if you have the willpower to combine breast-feeding with formula-feeding, there doesn't seem to be a biological reason why you can't do it. Meanwhile, plenty of women who have started off combination feeding, perhaps for medical reasons while in the hospital, have managed to switch to exclusive breast-feeding afterward—it just takes extra effort to get the milk supply going.

One final word of warning: Most experts agree that regular breast-feeding is essential in order to maintain the milk supply. So although giving babies the odd bottle of formula seems unlikely to make much difference to either their health or your ability to continue breast-feeding, regularly skipping breast feeds will cause the milk supply to diminish.

. 109 .
What is in formula milk, and why does it taste fishy?

All basic infant formula is made from cows' milk, although the proportions of the two main milk proteins, casein and whey, have been adjusted to mimic that of human milk more closely. Surprisingly, there's no difference between formula and breast milk in terms of the number of calories they provide, with both containing around 20 calories per ounce.

Many manufacturers produce formulas targeted at different age ranges. In "first milk" formulas, relatively more whey protein has been added, which makes it easier to digest. Formula marketed at "hungry babies" contains less whey and more casein, making it closer in composition to regular cows' milk. The idea is that casein forms a solid curd in the stomach and therefore takes longer to digest—which means, theoretically, the stomach stays fuller for longer—but it contains no more calories than normal formula and usually contains less fat. Nor is there any convincing evidence that babies are any less hungry on it, although they may be more likely to get constipated.

The same is true of "nighttime" milks, which contain starch to thicken them. The UK's Scientific Advisory Committee on Nutrition (SACN) recently published a statement saying there is no evidence that these offer any advantage over normal formula in terms of settling babies at night.

Meanwhile, "follow-on" formula (for older infants and toddlers) is usually marketed at babies aged six months and up, and it contains more iron, vitamin C, vitamin E, zinc, and calcium than normal formula. Most babies are eating at least some solid food by this stage so will be getting additional nutrients from that. Iron is also more readily absorbed from solid food than formula. The SACN has advised that there is no need to use follow-on milk instead of normal formula or cows' milk once babies reach one year of age. The American Academy of Pediatrics says that follow-on formulas offer no clear advantage over infant formulas designed to meet all nutritional needs over the first year, so you may as well let price guide you.

There's little difference between brands of basic formula in terms of their nutritional content. In the U.S. and Europe, at least, the use of the term "infant formula" is regulated, and all must meet minimum nutritional requirements. All are fortified with iron, which may be what gives formula a slightly metallic or fishy taste.

Some companies have started adding extra ingredients to basic formula, often alongside claims that these will boost babies' health:

Long-chain polyunsaturated fatty acids

Fatty acids such as docosahexaenoic acid (DHA) and arachidonic acid (AA) are added with the claim that they promote eye and brain development. Several recent studies have supported these claims—at least when higher doses of DHA and AA are added (so each comprises at least 0.3 percent of total fatty acids)—although others have found no benefit. A review by the Cochrane Collaboration showed no clear and consistent benefit of adding fatty acids to formula in terms of eye or brain development, or physical growth in healthy babies who weren't born prematurely.

Prebiotics and oligosaccharides

Another recent addition to formula milk is so-called prebiotics, or oligosaccharides (such as GOS or FOS). These are complex sugars found in breast milk and are thought to promote the growth of certain bacteria in the gut. A recent review concluded that adding them did increase the number of "friendly" bifidobacteria in the gut, and babies had softer and more frequent stools. However, a Cochrane review found no convincing evidence that prebiotics helped prevent allergies or food hypersensitivity, as some have claimed.

Probiotics

These are live bacteria that are sometimes added to formula milk. There is fairly strong evidence that probiotic supplements can reduce the development of eczema in babies with a strong family history of it.

Nucleotides

These form the basis of the DNA in every cell and are added to most formula these days. There is some evidence that they may reduce the incidence of diarrhea and boost response to vaccines, although many of these studies were funded by formula manufacturers, and other studies have found no effect. Given that most formulas contain nucleotides, and the jury is out on whether they have much benefit, it's probably not something to worry about.

Lactose-free or hypoallergenic formulas

Doctors sometimes recommend that babies with suspected feeding intolerances, such as lactase deficiency or milk-protein allergy, be fed a lactose-free or hypoallergenic formula. Pediatricians have voiced concerns that such conditions are being overdiagnosed and point out that spitting up milk is fairly normal, not necessarily an indication of an allergy or intolerance. These specialized formulas contain carbohydrates from corn or sucrose, rather than the carbohydrate found in milk called lactose. Hypoallergenic formula has also been treated with enzymes to break down the casein protein, against which some babies develop an immune reaction.

Soy formula

This is popular among parents who think it will be more digestible and less likely to trigger an allergic reaction, but a Cochrane review found that there wasn't enough evidence to recommend soy formula for prevention of allergy or food intolerance in babies at high risk of these conditions. Concerns have been raised about phytoestrogens in soy milk mimicking the female hormone estrogen. The European Society for Paediatric Gastroenterology, Hepatology, and Nutrition (ESPGHAN) recommends that soy formula be used only in babies older than six months who have been formally diagnosed with an allergy to milk protein.

. 110 .
Does "nipple confusion" really exist?

Parents are often told to avoid giving their baby a bottle or pacifier during the first three to four weeks of life, as it will cause nipple confusion. The idea is that the sucking action of breast-feeding differs from the technique used to extract milk from a bottle, so babies may become confused about how to breast-feed and even reject the breast as a result. Some claim that just one bottle feed can cause nipple confusion and that this might result in failure to establish breast-feeding. Yet many women physically can't breast-feed their newborn baby in the immediate aftermath of birth, so milk has to be given some other way. Traditionally, hospitals used bottles containing either expressed breast milk or formula, but fears about nipple confusion have led them to use a cup or feeding tube instead.

It's generally true that moms who start off mixing breast and bottle milk are less likely to continue breast-feeding, but the silicone teat isn't necessarily to blame. Alison Holmes and her colleagues at Dartmouth Medical School in New Hampshire studied 802 mother/baby pairs in which the baby had a combination of breast- and bottle-feeding during the first week in the hospital. Although such combination feeding shortened the amount of time that white babies were breast-fed, this was not the case for Latino or black babies. While it's possible that black and Hispanic babies are biologically different from white babies, this seems improbable. More likely is that the use of a silicone teat was irrelevant, and the white women were giving up breast-feeding for different reasons, possibly because they expected it to be a struggle after bottle-feeding and this then became a self-fulfilling prophecy. By contrast, Hispanic women have a strong tradition of combining breast- and bottle-feeding and see it as completely normal (see 108: "Could combining breast- and formula-feeding offer babies the best of both worlds?").

In a separate study, the Cochrane Collaboration reviewed four trials comparing cup- and bottle-feeding of breast milk to newborn babies. Although three of the studies found that the cup-fed infants were slightly more likely to be breast-fed exclusively when they were discharged from the hospital, there was no difference in the rate of exclusive breast-feeding when the babies were compared at the ages of three and six months. One of the studies suggested that cup-fed infants spent an average of ten days longer in the hospital than bottle-fed infants.

More evidence against the existence of nipple confusion comes from studies of the use of pacifiers by young babies. Although some studies have found a link between pacifier use and mothers giving up on breast-feeding, these couldn't show that the pacifiers themselves were to blame. What's more, several studies that combined the results of multiple clinical trials investigating the link between breast-feeding and pacifier use found that, when used in healthy breast-feeding babies, pacifiers had no significant effect on the proportion still breast-feeding at three months (see 97: "Are pacifiers good or bad for babies?").

. 111 .
Does what I eat change the flavor of my milk?

You might assume that an exclusive diet of milk would get rather boring after a while, but human milk provides a cornucopia of different flavor combinations that might even influence a baby's food preferences in later life. One of the most famous examples is carrots, as one study found that children whose mothers drank carrot juice during pregnancy or while breast-feeding showed a preference for carrot-flavored cereal (see 7: "Can Mom's food fads influence her baby's palate?").

In a separate study, breast-feeding moms were given edible capsules containing the same compounds that provided caraway seed, menthol, banana, and licorice their flavors. Although these flavors took varying amounts of time to show up in breast milk, appear they did. After just one hour, the milk took on the flavor of bananas, while after two hours, it began to taste of caraway and licorice. Menthol got into the milk after about two hours and stayed there for a further six hours. All four flavors disappeared eight hours after the capsules were eaten. However, there was considerable variation among the women in how the flavors were transferred to milk. If you suspect that something you've eaten may be upsetting your baby's delicate palate, eight hours should be long enough for any unpleasant flavors to be eliminated, says Helene Hausner at the University of Copenhagen in Denmark, who led the study.

Hausner has also found that different brands of formula milk vary in taste, so if your baby doesn't seem to like one brand, try another. Different brands generally have the same basic nutritional content.

. 112 .
How much alcohol gets into breast milk?

You've gone through nine months of abstinence during pregnancy and are just looking forward to enjoying wine with dinner again when a well-meaning friend asks, "Should you really be drinking if you're breast-feeding?" However, one midwife assured me that drinking actually aided breast-feeding by making you more relaxed and stimulating the milk-letdown reflex. Whom should you believe?

The fact is that alcohol does get into breast milk in about the same quantities as you would find in the blood, but it isn't stored there. So long as you wait to clear the alcohol from your system before breast-feeding, then your baby won't be exposed to it at all.

On a practical level, this means that if you were to drink an entire bottle of wine in the evening (about nine units, although wines vary in alcohol content), it would take around nine hours for this alcohol to leave your body, which means that you could breast-feed the following morning without having to worry about it. And because alcohol isn't stored in the breasts, there's no need to pump out the residual milk and pour it down the drain.

It's also a relief to know that a toxic-breakdown product of alcohol called acetaldehyde—which is partly responsible for hangover symptoms such as headaches and vomiting—doesn't pass into breast milk. And even if you decided to breast-feed immediately after having a drink, the alcohol that your baby received would be greatly diluted as a result of passing through your body. In the 1980s, researchers from New Zealand encouraged eight nursing mothers to drink as much alcohol as they could manage in as short a time as possible, and then measured how much of it they could detect in the milk. They found that the alcohol level in blood and milk peaked between one and a half to two hours after drinking and then began to fall; even at the peak, the amounts were far less than would have been present in the original drink. For example, the researchers calculated that if a six-month-old baby weighing around 14 pounds drank 6 ounces of milk when its mother's blood alcohol content was .19 percent (the legal U.S. limit is .08 percent), the baby's blood alcohol level would rise to just .006 percent. Although babies have less of the enzyme that breaks down alcohol than adults, "It is improbable that occasional exposure to alcohol of that quantity would affect the child," writes Margaret Lawton of the Department of Scientific and Industrial Research in Auckland, who led the research.

Although there's no current evidence to suggest that such tiny amounts of alcohol cause any lasting damage to babies, it may have subtle effects on their behavior. For example, Julie Mennella of the Monell Chemical Senses Center in Philadelphia has been studying the transfer of alcohol into breast milk for over two decades and has found that just one to two alcoholic drinks will change the flavor of breast milk. Babies are thought to learn about flavors through drinking breast milk, so it is possible that regular drinking may have an influence on their taste for alcohol in the future. In the short term, at least, Mennella has found that the babies of moms who regularly enjoy a drink while breast-feeding seem to be more interested in chewing a toy that smells of alcohol than if their mother abstains.

Consuming alcoholic breast milk may also affect the quality of a baby's sleep. In a small study, Mennella gave babies 3.4 ounces of breast milk flavored with 2 teaspoons of alcohol, the sort of amount they'd receive if their mothers had been drinking heavily. She found that the babies tended to fall asleep faster but slept for significantly shorter periods of time in the three and a half hours after drinking the alcoholic milk compared to when they drank pure breast milk. "Babies have less active sleep and then compensate for it in the next few days if Mom doesn't drink again," says Mennella. She adds that similar changes in sleep patterns have been seen in older fetuses whose mothers drink during the latter stages of pregnancy.

Finally, Mennella has blown the lid on the received wisdom that a glass of wine helps to stimulate the milk-letdown reflex. In fact, alcohol blocks the release of oxytocin, leading to an overall reduction in milk production. Mennella found that babies consumed 20 percent less breast milk on average in the three to four hours after their mothers had been drinking, compared with babies whose mothers hadn't had an alcoholic drink. What's more, they seemed to increase the intensity of their sucking and the number of times they demanded a feed in the next eight to twelve hours, in order to compensate—not necessarily what you want when you're suffering from a hangover. The mothers who drank noticed that their breasts felt fuller, which may be the origin of the myth that alcohol increases milk production.

. 113 .
Is morning breast milk any different from evening breast milk?

In 2009, Spanish researchers made a fascinating discovery: Breast milk produced during the evening appears to contain natural sedatives that may promote drowsiness. These chemicals (called nucleotides) play other important roles within cells, but several have been implicated in the processes of sleep.

Cristina Sánchez at the University of Extremadura in Badajoz, Spain, looked at levels of the three nucleotides most strongly linked to sleep in the milk of thirty breast-feeding women over the course of twenty-four hours. She found that levels of a nucleotide called 5´AMP (adenosine monophosphate) were highest in the evening, while levels of 5´GMP (guanosine monophosphate) and 5´UMP (uridine monophosphate) increased as the night wore on. All were found at far lower concentrations during the daytime.

The most likely explanation is that 5´AMP in breast milk stimulates the release of another sleep-promoting chemical in the brain called GABA, while

5´GMP fuels the production of melatonin, which helps to regulate the body's natural clock. 5´UMP is known to promote both REM and non-REM sleep. These are early findings, but they at least hint that babies given a nighttime feed of formula or breast milk expressed during the day won't be getting this natural sleep aid.

Night feeds may have some sleep benefits for moms too. Breast-feeding activates the release of a hormone called prolactin, which promotes drowsiness and increases the relative proportion of deep sleep. This is the kind of sleep that refreshes you and leaves you ready to tackle the next day. A small study found that women who breast-fed their babies spent more time in deep sleep and less in light sleep compared to those who bottle-fed their infants, even though they spent a similar amount of time awake. One implication might be that night feeds have less of an impact on women who breast-feed because they get more good-quality deep sleep to compensate.

. 114 .
Can men lactate?

Many fathers envy the closeness that breast-feeding brings, while I'm sure many moms wish at certain points that their partner could share the job of feeding.

Men actually possess all of the equipment needed to breast-feed, including milk ducts and mammary tissue; they just don't produce enough of the hormones to trigger milk production under normal circumstances. One of the main hormones involved in breast-feeding is prolactin, which new fathers are known to produce in small quantities and which seems to stimulate paternal behavior (see 32: "Do men change when they become dads?").

Prolactin is produced by the pituitary gland, and men who develop pituitary tumors sometimes lactate. Certain drugs, including the antipsychotic drug Thorazine and the heart drug digoxin, can stimulate milk production in men, as can a medical condition called galactorrhea, in which the nipples begin to leak a milky discharge. Galactorrhea is associated with high levels of prolactin and low levels of testosterone.

Intriguingly, this "male milk" seems to be similar in composition to that produced by women. In 1981, researchers at the University of Western Australia tested the nipple secretions of a twenty-seven-year-old man with galactorrhea and found in it levels of protein, sugar, and electrolytes comparable to those in female breast milk and colostrum.

Unfortunately, I've failed in my attempts to convince my husband that he should try pumping his breasts or taking hormone supplements to see if any milk comes out. If anyone else succeeds, please let me know!

Weaning

. 115 .
When should I wean my baby on to solid foods?

Just a decade ago, parents were told to start introducing solid foods from four months of age. Then, in 2002, the World Health Organization brought out guidelines saying that babies should be exclusively breast-fed for six months and solids could be introduced after that. The main reason given was that breast-feeding provides some protection against infection, and the more breast milk babies receive, the greater the level of protection (see 106: "Is breast really best for babies?").

Two months is a long time in the life of a baby, and this change has left some parents in a state of confusion. Does it mean that introducing solids earlier than six months is bad for babies? And what should parents do if their baby is formula-fed?

The consensus among pediatricians is that starting solids before the age of four months is a bad idea. Different studies have shown an increase in symptoms of asthma, eczema, and obesity among children given solids before four months. However, the evidence is by no means clear-cut: A separate review of five studies conducted in the UK found no difference in the health of babies given solids at the age of twelve weeks.

Once babies reach four months, the picture gets even fuzzier. Both the

American Academy of Pediatrics and the European Society for Paediatric Gastroenterology, Hepatology, and Nutrition say that solid foods can be introduced between four and six months of age.

One reason parents might want to start introducing solids before six months is because they think that their baby needs the extra nutrients, or that it will help them sleep longer at night. Although the UK review found that breast-fed babies were more likely to be sleeping through the night if given solids at twelve weeks of age, other studies have found no difference in sleep patterns between early- and late-weaned babies.

Meanwhile, at least one good-quality study in the U.S. found no advantage in starting solids early in terms of a baby's overall growth. By the age of twelve months, formula-fed babies weighed and measured the same, regardless of whether solids were introduced at three or six months, and their bodies contained a similar proportion of fat and muscle. Even though they drank slightly less milk, the overall number of calories the babies consumed was roughly the same, suggesting that babies are able to regulate the amount they eat according to how hungry they are.

Other arguments in favor of introducing early solids include exposing babies to a wide range of flavors so they're less likely to become picky eaters, and rumors that babies will experience feeding problems if they don't learn to chew before six months of age. There's little evidence to support either of these claims, and a good-quality trial from Honduras found no difference in appetite or food acceptance between breast-fed babies given solids at either four or six months of age.

On the other hand, at least one study has found that waiting to introduce solids until six months reduced the risk of asthma in babies with a family history of allergies. It's also true that babies are less likely to encounter bacteria that could make them sick if they continue to be fed milk rather than solid food.

Overall, it seems there's little benefit in introducing solids before six months, especially if you're breast-feeding. If nothing else, weaning can be hard work because it requires extra levels of organization and preparation. But if you do start after four months—particularly if your baby is showing a strong interest—there's scant evidence that it will do any harm.

. 116 .
How do I get my baby to like vegetables?

Many babies naturally shy away from bitter flavors such as those found in certain vegetables, but if your baby initially rejects broccoli or spinach, don't despair. Feeding children a range of different vegetables may be enough to get them used to the overall taste, ultimately resulting in the acceptance of the scorned vegetable.

Julie Mennella and her colleagues at the Monell Chemical Senses Center in Philadelphia took seventy-four babies aged between four and nine months with at least two weeks' experience of eating cereals or fruit and split them into two groups. The first was introduced to pureed green beans, while the remaining babies were given pureed pear. All of the babies were assessed on how well they accepted this new flavor.

Over the next eight days, the babies were subdivided. In the bean group, some babies were given green beans to eat every dinnertime, while others were given a different vegetable at each dinner. Still others were given a variety of vegetables both within and between meals. A similar strategy was employed with the pear group, introducing a mixture of different fruits instead of vegetables. After the eight days were up, both groups were given pears or green beans to taste once more. Although all the babies ate more of the original fruit or vegetable than they did the first time around, babies who had been eating a wide variety of different fruits or vegetables during the week showed the greatest increase in the amount of pear or green bean they consumed.

Mennella thinks that repeatedly exposing babies to lots of different flavors from the same overall food group may teach them to be more accepting of individual flavors within that group. She suggests persevering even if babies grimace when they are eating the food; the important thing is that they are getting a taste of it. Other studies have hinted that babies need to taste a food eight to ten times before they willingly start to accept it—although forcing babies to eat something they don't want can result in a long-term aversion to it.

If this strategy doesn't work, you could try mixing the offending food with something the baby does like. Although this hasn't been tested in very young babies, Elizabeth Capaldi of Arizona State University in Tempe has shown that children from two to five can be taught to like the sour taste of grapefruit juice by having it mixed with sugar the first few times they try it. Importantly, they go on liking unsweetened grapefruit juice when they taste it again, even after a gap of several weeks. If all else fails, show your baby pictures of the food you want him to eat beforehand. Several studies have suggested that toddlers are more likely to try a new fruit or vegetable if they have seen it in a book. A copy of *The Very Hungry Caterpillar* should definitely be at the top of any picky eater's reading list!

. 117 .
Is there any evidence for baby-led weaning being better than parent-led weaning?

The first taste of food is a rite of passage for any baby (and excited parent). But quite aside from the debate about when to introduce it, the other big question is how. One current trend is to ditch spoon-fed purees in favor of baby-led weaning, encouraging babies to self-feed from the outset.

In its purest form, this means no spoon-feeding whatsoever. Babies eat what they fancy, and if that's nothing, then fine. But a baby on food strike can be a source of enormous anxiety to new parents, particularly as few of us have any clue as to how much they should be eating (see 119: "How many calories does a baby need?"). Self-feeding can also be an extremely messy affair, and many parents worry that young babies will choke if given chunks of food rather than easy-to-swallow purees.

I had no choice: Our daughter, Matilda, refused to let a spoon pass her lips unless she was controlling it (or it contained fruit yogurt). Since she wasn't adept at levering food onto a spoon (and no baby can live on YoBaby alone), this meant that finger foods such as toast, scrambled eggs, pasta, fruit, and vegetables were her main source of solids in the early days.

Is one method any better than the other? Baby-led weaning is a relatively new phenomenon, so unfortunately, there's very little research to draw on, although in 2012, British researchers published a study comparing the eating habits of 155 children aged twenty months to six and a half years who had been introduced to solids through either spoon-feeding or baby-led weaning. Key questions included what they liked to eat now, how picky they were, and how much they weighed.

In general, children introduced to solids through baby-led weaning had a stronger preference for carbohydrates than the spoon-fed children, who liked sweet foods best. The baby-led group also had a lower body mass index on average than the spoon-fed group, although there was no difference in the number of picky eaters between the two groups.

One flaw of this study is that it relied on parents reporting what their children ate rather than measuring it directly. We also don't know how strict they were about the weaning process (as many parents who spoon-feed also give their children finger foods to eat) or at what age they started weaning.

Most advocates of baby-led weaning suggest waiting until the baby is six months old before introducing solid food, as before this, babies may not possess the coordination to grasp food, chew it, and swallow it. But there's fairly unanimous agreement that from six months, babies start needing the extra nutrients that solids provide, so a key question is whether all babies are developmentally ready to start eating finger foods at this age.

In a separate study, another team of British researchers investigated the age at which babies started reaching out for food. Six hundred and two parents were interviewed when their baby was eight months old. Of these, just over half said their child had started reaching for food before the age of six months; 6 percent still were not reaching out for food at the age of eight months. Asked whether their babies were now eating finger foods, over 90 percent said they ate some at least daily, although 35 percent were described as needing to be fully fed at mealtimes.

American studies also hint that some babies may not be ready to eat finger foods by six months. One study found that 68 percent of four- to six-month-olds had begun grasping foods, but just 53 percent of seven- to eight-month-olds could eat food that needed chewing.

The message I take away is that it comes down to the individual baby. If they your child seems ready to start eating finger foods at six months, great, but there's currently no strong evidence to suggest that offering a mixture of finger foods and purees is any less good. It's also pretty clear that some babies won't be ready to eat finger foods at six months, so, given that they do start needing some solids from this age, it's probably wise to spoon-feed them until they are ready to self-feed.

If you decide to try baby-led weaning, you may find that mealtimes take longer, although this isn't necessarily grounds for concern. Another study showed that fifteen-month-olds eating a finger-fed meal took around twice as long to eat half as much food as during a spoon-fed meal, but the average number of calories they consumed was the same. This is because finger foods such as toast, cheese, and pasta tend to be denser than when food is fed as a puree.

. 118 .
Should I force my baby to eat?

One thing baby-led weaning has in its favor is an altogether more relaxed attitude to food and feeding. In a study of 702 mothers, those following the baby-led approach reported feeling less pressure to get their child to eat and seemed less concerned about their baby's weight than women who were spoon-feeding their babies. The same study found no association between weaning style and the baby's weight.

Regardless of how you choose to feed your baby, a relaxed approach is important, since a domineering attitude to mealtimes can have a negative impact on a baby's weight and eating habits as it grows older. Studies in children over the age of one have shown that pressuring them to eat increases pickiness, fussiness, and the risk of them being underweight, while restricting access to certain foods often results in them eating more of that food when the opportunity does arise.

Although it is less well studied, parental attitude seems to affect younger babies' eating habits, too. One study of six-month-olds who had been slow to put on weight found that babies whose moms had a relaxed approach to feeding put on significantly more weight in the following six months than those whose moms had a controlling attitude to food. The converse was true in babies who were heavier than average at six months. Left to their own devices, it seems that babies will eventually respond to their body's needs and regulate their food intake appropriately.

. 119 .
How many calories does a baby need?

Few parents think about the number of calories babies are consuming when all they're drinking is milk, but weaning can bring on a whole new set of anxieties. I remember worrying about my daughter having eaten only a single spoon of pea puree (despite drinking plenty of milk), and trying to fill her up on banana—a taste she definitely liked.

Just how many calories a baby needs depends on its size and age, but as a general rule, very young babies need around 110 calories per kilogram (a kilogram is about 2.2 pounds) per day—so a one-month-old weighing four and a half kilograms (10 pounds) would need around 495 calories (all from milk).

As babies get older, their rate of growth slows, so the number of calories they need per pound of body weight begins to fall. By the age of six months (when most babies start eating solid food), it has dropped to around 80 calories per kilogram (36 calories per pound) per day, and it hovers around this point for the rest of the first year. This means that a six-month-old weighing seven and a half kilograms (16.5 pounds) would need around 600 calories per day, some of which it will get from milk and the rest from solid food. Both breast- and formula-milk contain around 20 calories per ounce, so if a six-month-old is drinking 20 ounces of milk per day (400 calories), it needs only an extra 200 calories from solid food. That's not very much: equivalent to approximately two bananas.

A one-year-old weighing 22 pounds will need around 800 calories per day, and its milk consumption probably will have dropped by now. Assuming he's drinking around 15 ounces of cows' milk per day, which contains 270 calories (there are 18 calories per ounces of whole cows' milk), this would mean he needs an extra 530 calories from solid food. That's still only about a quarter to a fifth of what the average adult should be consuming in a day.

Of course, individual babies vary in appetite, and there may be some days when they are hungrier or less hungry. The best measure of whether a baby is eating enough is whether it is maintaining a healthy weight.

. 120 .
Should I avoid feeding my baby nuts or eggs to protect it against allergies?

Some parents worry about introducing foods such as eggs, fish, or nuts into a baby's diet for fear that it might increase the risk of developing allergies or eczema. Although there is some evidence to support this, plenty of studies have found no effect, while some even suggest that the early introduction of such foods can have a protective effect.

It's quite true that allergens from foods such as nuts and eggs can find their way into breast milk. For this reason, the American Academy of Pediatrics (AAP) used to tell mothers whose babies were at high risk of allergy to avoid feeding eggs until they were two years of age, and to avoid fish and nuts until they were three.

However, as more studies have been published, this advice has changed, and the current scientific consensus is that there's no reason to avoid such foods during breast-feeding or weaning. In its most recent statement, the AAP said that the current evidence does not support women avoiding certain food groups during pregnancy or breast-feeding, and there's little evidence that delaying the introduction of foods such as fish, eggs, and those that contain peanuts prevents allergy, asthma, or eczema.

European experts seem to agree. The European Society for Paediatric Gastroenterology, Hepatology, and Nutrition recently reviewed the evidence and concluded that, in general, solids should be introduced after seventeen weeks and no later than twenty-six weeks, adding that there is no convincing scientific evidence that avoiding fish and eggs reduces allergies, even in high-risk babies. It cautions against introducing gluten (which is found in wheat) before four months or after seven months of age, and advises to do so gradually, as there's some evidence that this strategy reduces the risk of celiac disease, type 1 diabetes, and wheat allergy.

It's fine to add small quantities of cows' milk to food, although that shouldn't be the main source of milk before the age of one, as they can't absorb enough iron from it.

The Brown Stuff

. 121 .
Are reusable diapers really greener than disposables?

Many eco-conscious parents shared a sigh of relief when in 2005 the UK's Environment Agency announced that disposable diapers were no worse for the environment than reusable ones. Disposable diapers account for around 2.4 percent of the household waste that ends up as landfill in the UK, and few parents like the thought of bags of dirty diapers clogging up the countryside for hundreds of years (even if they are buried underground). Their degradation also produces methane, a potent greenhouse gas. However, laundering reusable diapers also takes an environmental toll, as energy is needed to fuel the washing machines that get them clean.

The Environment Agency concluded that neither type of diaper could claim environmental superiority. To put it in context, over the average two and a half years that a baby is in diapers, both are roughly comparable with driving a car between 1,300 and 2,200 miles in terms of greenhouse-gas emissions and depletion of nonrenewable resources.

The U.S.-based Union of Concerned Scientists has similarly advised parents not to waste a great deal of time or energy trying to weigh the environmental impact of the different types of diapers, because the differences aren't particularly dramatic. In its recently published *Consumers' Guide to Effective*

Environmental Choices, the union suggests opting for cloth diapers if you live somewhere with shortages in landfill space, and disposable diapers if you live somewhere plagued by water shortages.

There are some circumstances in which cloth diapers can be greener. In 2008, the Environment Agency released an updated report concluding that the eco-credentials of reusable diapers varied widely according to how they were washed. Disposable and reusable diapers might produce similar greenhouse-gas emissions based on average washer and tumble-dryer use, but washing reusable diapers in fuller loads or line-drying the diapers outdoors reduced emissions by 16 percent, making them less damaging than disposables. If you did this and used the diapers for a second child, this would cut the environmental impact by 40 percent (although this is still only equivalent to driving some 620 miles by car). In contrast, if parents tumble-dried all their reusable diapers, this would increase their environmental impact by 43 percent, while washing diapers at 90°C (194°F) instead of at 60°C (140°F) would increase it by 31 percent.

In other words, you can cut the environmental impact of diapers by using reusable ones—so long as you're prepared to wait until you have a full load of wash, wash them at 120 to 140°F in an energy-efficient machine, and leave them to dry naturally.

What about the effect of different diapers on the health of babies' bottoms? According to a recent review of twenty-eight different studies by the Cochrane Collaboration, there is little good-quality evidence to say that either type of diaper is any better than another in terms of preventing diaper rash. Studies looking at differences in scrotal temperatures between young boys wearing disposable or reusable diapers have also produced mixed results, so any claims that disposables might affect boys' later fertility should also, for now, be regarded with skepticism.

. 122 .
What about eco-friendly disposables?

Not all disposable diapers are equal, at least if you believe the packaging. There are regular diapers, and then there are eco-friendly biodegradable diapers. I know plenty of moms who have opted for the eco-friendly option in a bid to assuage their guilt about not using cloth diapers, but does it make much difference?

It depends on which bit of "environmentally friendly" you care most about. In terms of greenhouse-gas emissions, there is little direct evidence to support the use of biodegradable disposables over regular ones. In fact, unless you plan to compost your diapers, placing a biodegradable diaper in a dustbin is a pretty futile exercise—and could make things worse.

Bambo Nature, an Australian company that claims its diapers are 75 percent biodegradable, admits that throwing them in the regular dustbin won't cause them to biodegrade: "Any nappy that claims to be biodegradable only biodegrades if it is composted, not if it is thrown into landfill," says its website. This is because garbage in landfill is usually cut off from the water, oxygen, and bacteria needed for decomposition to occur.

"We think that things should biodegrade in landfill, but we've taken excruciating steps to prevent them from interacting with the natural environment because, traditionally, landfills have had major problems with the contamination of groundwater," says Adam Gendell of the U.S. organization GreenBlue, which promotes sustainability to businesses.

Even food waste and grass cuttings struggle to decompose fully in landfill, and although some newer biodegradable diapers contain chemicals designed to speed up the breakdown of the plastics they contain, this process releases methane, which is bad for the environment.

In an ideal world, it would be better if nothing went to landfill, because many of the things we throw away could be recycled or composted. "But if we do have to send some things to landfill, and I imagine that used diapers will be one of the last holdouts of things that do, then it's okay for them not to biodegrade," says Gendell.

If you want to try to compost your biodegradable diapers, Bambo recommends only home composting, not sending them to communal facilities. Even then, some of the plastic parts will not biodegrade and will need to be manually removed.

Of course, there are other environmental considerations besides greenhouse-gas emissions and biodegradability. Unbleached diapers use fewer harmful chemicals in their manufacture, and diapers containing wood from sustainably sourced forests clearly have better eco-credentials than those that don't. The greenest option of all is using cloth diapers (washed at a moderate temperature and left to dry naturally) and then reusing them on a second or third baby.

. 123 .
Why is baby poop yellow?

The color of poop is influenced mostly by two pigments, bilirubin and biliverdin, both breakdown products of red blood cells. Bilirubin starts off as a yellowish pigment but is further broken down and oxidized into a brown pigment called stercobilin, while biliverdin is green. Mix them together and you end up with the characteristic brown of feces, but as in a child's paint box, the final shade depends on how much of these pigments gets added to the mix.

The key factor that determines the final color of poop is how long it takes to travel through the digestive system. If it travels extremely quickly, it will be green; if it takes a bit longer, the color becomes yellow; while slower stools tend to be brown.

Breast milk is very easy to digest, so it slips through the digestive system quickly. This means very little pigment is added, and the bilirubin doesn't have time to get converted into stercobilin, hence the yellow color of breast-fed babies' poop. If a baby isn't getting enough of the creamy hindmilk at the end of a feed, the milk will travel through the system even faster, often resulting in watery green poop and gas, caused by fermentation of undigested protein in the lower intestines (see 89: "What causes colic?"). Formula-fed babies produce a rainbow of different shades from green to brown, depending on the composition of the formula (see 109: "What is in formula milk, and why does it taste fishy?").

Apart from the tar-black meconium you might notice in your newborn's first couple of diapers, babies' poop shouldn't be black. If it is, this may be a sign of internal bleeding, as are streaks of red in the stools. Meconium isn't really poop at all; rather than consisting of digested food, it contains decomposed intestinal cells that have been sloughed off during the baby's development.

As you start to introduce solid food into your baby's diet, you will probably notice stools becoming harder and browner. Certain foods can also leave unprepared parents with a fright: Beetroot and raspberries can result in various shades of red, while bananas can produce what look like black worms. Because of its high-fiber content, sweet corn barely gets digested at all and comes out looking the same as it went in.

. 124 .
Why does baby poop smell like mustard?

Simple answer: because, like mustard, baby poop contains vinegar. Breast-fed babies tend to have yellow and fairly liquid stools, which smell very different than adult ones. The smell is influenced by the bacteria living in your bowels, and breast milk contains large amounts of indigestible carbohydrates called oligosaccharides, which foster the growth of bacteria called bifidobacteria and lactobacilli. When fermented, these oligosaccharides give rise to hydrogen gas and chemicals such as propionic acid, butyric acid, and acetic acid—or vinegar, as it is more commonly known.

"Oligosaccharides are also thought to be responsible for the short passage time and for the stools being soft-liquidish," says Ekhard Ziegler, a pediatrician at the University of Iowa who has studied gas production in breast- and formula-fed babies. Formula milk contains no oligosaccharides but larger amounts of sulfur-containing amino acids, which encourage the growth of Enterobacteriaceae—bacteria commonly found in adult intestines. Parents often comment that poop from formula-fed babies is stinkier, and this is because digested formula produces more sulfurous gases, such as hydrogen sulfide and methanethiol. Babies fed soy-based formula produce particularly large amounts of hydrogen sulfide, which smells of rotten eggs.

On a slight tangent, one study recently found that moms prefer the smell of their own baby's diapers compared to those of unrelated babies. One possibility is that they're more accustomed to their own child's smells (and blinded by love, of course). But since gut bacteria are passed from mother to baby during birth, it is also possible that their baby's poop smells more similar to their own.

. 125 .
Is baby poop "cleaner" than adult poop?

You know the scenario. Your baby's diaper explodes. Torrents of molten poop trickle out of the sides, over her clothes, and leak into her sheets. Then, halfway through being changed, your baby performs an alligator death roll and gets poo all over its feet and hair, not to mention you. But surely baby poop is "cleaner" than adult poop, and therefore slightly less revolting?

Not necessarily. Babies are born with sterile guts, meaning that for the first few days of life, there are few, if any, bacteria coming out of the other end. But that all changes pretty quickly, and by the end of the first month, there are approximately thirty trillion bacteria per fluid ounce of poop—about the same number as in adults. How do they get there? Babies gulp down mouthfuls of bacteria from their mother's vagina during birth and pick up still more from her skin and milk during breast-feeding. These travel down the esophagus, through the stomach, and set up camp in the intestines, where they grow and flourish. This colonization continues throughout life through the foods and drinks we consume; many of these bacteria perform useful functions such as helping us to digest food and keeping our immune systems healthy.

There is a difference in the types of bacteria found in the poop of babies and adults, with adults harboring a more complex range than newborns. But as solid food is introduced, the diversity of the bacteria increases until it stabilizes at around one to two years, when it reaches its adult composition— and this is as unique as a fingerprint.

The type of bacteria can vary according to how a baby was born and whether or not it was breast-fed. A study by John Penders and his colleagues at Maastricht University in the Netherlands found that babies who are born by C-section or formula-fed harbor more potentially harmful and less beneficial bacteria than breast-fed babies and those born naturally. This is because in a C-section, the first bacteria that babies are exposed to come from the hospital environment, rather than their mothers, while formula-fed babies acquire fewer bacteria from their mother's milk and skin.

While the vast majority of gut bacteria are helpful rather than harmful, both babies and adults carry potentially disease-causing bacteria in their guts, so you should always be sure to wash your hands after diaper-changing.

Baby Brains

Is the temperament of a newborn carried through into childhood and beyond?

Pretty soon after your baby is born, you'll realize it's far from being a blank slate and already has characteristics that distinguish it from other babies you know. Some are sleepy, others seem fascinated by new objects, while others are fussy and overreact to every situation they're placed in. Are these passing traits, or can they tell us something about the sort of people our babies will grow up to be?

Studies of twins have suggested that certain aspects of our personalities are at least partially inherited, including how emotional, active, social, and impulsive we are. These traits don't necessarily show up in infancy. When scientists talk about personality in young babies, they tend to refer to temperament—things such as the intensity of their emotions, how sensitive they are to their environment, and how easy they are to soothe. In other words, these are traits that emerge at an extremely young age and seem to be independent of experience, intelligence, or learning—a bit like the basic fabric of an artist's canvas. Personality, on the other hand, is who you are on top of your temperament—like the painting that goes on the canvas.

One suggestion is that many babies fall into one of three temperamental "types." Easy babies are generally cheerful and easy to calm, adjust quickly to new situations and routines, and have normal eating and sleeping patterns. Around 40 percent of babies are considered "easy." Difficult babies tend to be emotional, irritable, fussy, and cry a lot. They often have irregular eating and sleeping patterns. Around 10 percent of babies have "difficult" temperaments. Slow-to-warm babies are relatively inactive and tend to withdraw from new situations and people. Although they take time to adapt to new experiences, they do accept them eventually. Around 15 percent of babies are considered "slow to warm."

Not all babies fit neatly into one of these three boxes (which is why the percentages don't add up), and there's no guarantee that an easy baby will grow into an easy toddler, and so on. Temperament can change quite a lot during the first few months, since factors such as having experienced a difficult birth or being born prematurely can have temporary effects on babies' behavior.

There are some aspects of temperament that do seem to remain relatively consistent. One of the best studied is how babies react to unexpected situations. Although most babies are fascinated by new things and being taken out into new surroundings, around 15 percent of babies are described as "highly reactive," which means they tend to be easily distressed by new and unexpected events—possibly because they are easily overwhelmed by stimuli. One study found that highly reactive babies are more likely to have narrow faces, which might suggest some kind of genetic predisposition. Highly reactive babies can be hard work for parents: They fuss, cry, and need more soothing than other babies—to the extent that parents may feel as if they're being deliberately pushed away. As toddlers, highly reactive types tend to be slightly more shy and reserved, and there's some evidence that they grow into more introverted adults who are at higher risk of being worry-prone and anxious. On the plus side, they are more likely to focus on details and can be meticulous planners. But they're sensitive souls who need nurturing and are particularly vulnerable to the effects of bad parenting (see 128: "Can parents modify their baby's personality traits?").

Once a baby has passed the nine-month mark, some other aspects of temperament emerge that can give a hint of what parents can expect as their baby begins to blossom into a child. These include how quickly babies approach new objects—thought to be a measure of sociability and extroversion—and how fearful, angry, and active they are.

Fear

Although fear might sound like a negative quality, it is thought to play an important role in the development of conscience, because children are more worried about potential punishment. Fearful babies are less likely to grow into impulsive or aggressive children, but they may also be more prone to depression and loneliness.

Novelty

Happy babies who approach new objects rapidly have a tendency to grow into more extroverted and outgoing individuals, but they may also be more impulsive, show less self-control, and easily angered or frustrated.

Anger

Babies who show early signs of anger at around ten months seem to grow into active children with a positive outlook, but they can also be impulsive and easily angered or frustrated.

Activity

Active babies have a tendency to become active children, who are extroverted and open, but they can be disagreeable.

. 127 .
When do babies develop a sense of themselves as individuals?

Although some aspects of a baby's temperament become evident during the first year, other traits—such as pride, embarrassment, shame, and guilt—don't tend to emerge until babies begin to recognize themselves as "selves." This usually happens between eighteen months and two years of age, at around the same time they start to recognize their reflection in a mirror. You can test this on your own baby by sitting him in front of a mirror and seeing how he reacts to it. Babies younger than a year may reach toward the mirror or smile at it. Now try removing him and putting a small dot of lipstick or paint on the tip of his nose. After a short gap, put him back in front of the mirror and see how he reacts. If the baby is younger than around fifteen months, it's unlikely he'll do very much, but as babies get older, they begin to realize that that blob of color in the reflection relates to their own nose, and they'll try and wipe it off by reaching for their nose (rather than the reflection). This reaction becomes more common as babies reach eighteen months to two years.

Studies have shown that once babies start to recognize their reflections, they are more prone to showing embarrassment, as they realize that others also see them as individuals.

Between fifteen months and two years, babies start to use the personal pronouns "my" or "mine," prompting a flurry of claims on everything from your phone—"my phone"; to your wallet—"my wallet"; to the floor—"my floor." This is the start of babies beginning to recognize themselves as individuals, but it is a fairly lengthy process. Parents will notice that babies tend to be extremely reluctant to share, and like nothing better than to snatch a toy or instrument away from another child—leading to excruciating exchanges with other parents as you try to explain away your child's apparent selfishness. Although empathy and sharing may seem like obvious things to adults, they are possible only once you recognize the existence of two selves—one's self and another's self—each with an identity, needs, thoughts, and desires. This is also known as theory of mind. Precisely when this develops is still very much up for debate, but few researchers would argue that children have it much before the age of three, and some don't think it fully develops until children are five.

. 128 .
Can parents modify their baby's personality traits?

Let's assume your baby shows signs of being "highly reactive" (see 126: "Is the temperament of a newborn carried through into childhood and beyond?"), but you don't want her to grow into an anxious child. You shouldn't worry too much, because parents still have a massive impact on the type of person their baby grows up to be.

Let's take a Dutch study that found that babies deemed to be highly reactive or irritable when they were fifteen days old were less likely to be securely attached at the age of one. Secure attachment is a reflection of how "bonded" a baby is to its mother or main caregiver, and babies who are insecurely attached show little preference for that caregiver over a complete stranger.

The researchers found that moms of irritable babies interacted with them less and were less likely to notice when their babies were giving them positive signals about wanting to play or be cuddled than the mothers of nonirritable infants. However, if the same researchers gave the moms advice on how to comfort and play with their babies, they found that these babies were just as likely to have formed secure attachments by the age of one as nonirritable babies. This suggests that how parents respond to a baby's temperamental traits can play a huge role in how they develop. An irritable baby may be harder to soothe and may push its mother away, but if a mother pays attention to its needs and provides comfort when it is unhappy, it will flourish just like any other child.

The culture in which a child is raised may play a big role in how different temperaments play out in later life. One study that compared how Canadian and Chinese mothers responded to shyness in their children found that, whereas Chinese mothers approved of shyness, Canadian moms saw it as a negative trait and tried to draw the children out of their shells. A later study by the same group found cultural differences in the way peers reacted to a shy child. Canadian four-year-olds tended to reject shy classmates, while Chinese children seemed to like them. Perhaps it's no wonder that Chinese people are often more restrained than Westerners.

. 129 .

Does the order of birth influence children's personalities?

Are firstborns such as Bill Clinton and Tony Blair ambitious yet conventional because they're firstborns? Perhaps Bill Gates and Ricky Gervais are helpful and sociable because they're middle children, and Charles Darwin and Mozart were creative and rebellious because, as younger siblings, they felt the need to stand out.

The extent to which order of birth affects personality is a debate that has been raging among psychologists for several decades. A number of studies have suggested that firstborns tend to be more achievement-oriented, conscientious, hardworking, organized, and reliable than later-born children, while later-born children are generally more extroverted, open to new experiences, and agreeable than firstborns. The latest research suggests that when it comes to certain attributes, there may be some truth to this thinking, even if much that has been written on birth order is flawed.

Although most parents believe they raise siblings in exactly the same way, the research contradicts that. Studies of identical twins have found that certain attributes of their personalities, such as intelligence, are up to 70 percent genetic. However, if twins are split up and raised in separate families, studies have found that their social attitudes and interests, as well as personality traits such as how aggressive or impulsive they are, are no more different than if they had been raised in the same family. In other words, growing up in the same family doesn't have a great deal of impact in terms of making siblings resemble each other. This suggests that parents respond to siblings as individuals, even if they are twins.

One reason why much of the research on birth order has been criticized is that it hasn't taken the size of people's families into account. If most of the firstborns who are studied come from small families or are only children, then they're likely to have had very different upbringings from second- or third-born children from large families, regardless of when in the order of siblings they were born.

However, several recent studies don't suffer from this problem, and they provide at least some support for the idea that birth order makes a difference—albeit a small one.

For example, in 2009, Joshua Hartshorne and his colleagues at Harvard University found that people tend to associate with those who are in a similar position in the family pecking order, so firstborns are more likely to befriend other firstborns, and so on. Since other studies have shown that we tend to be attracted to people with similar personality traits, this is at least indirect evidence that birth order might shape our personalities to some degree. Birth order may also have an impact on intelligence. Petter Kristensen and his colleagues at Oslo University studied the military records of 241,310 Norwegian conscripts and found that, on average, eldest children had higher IQs than second-born children. It wasn't a big difference—just 2.3 points on the IQ scale—but it might be enough to put someone at the top of the class rather than the middle (and this might have other knock-on effects in terms of confidence or how hard a child is pushed to work). Interestingly, it didn't seem to come down to having been born first but to being raised as the elder child. Kristensen found that those who took on the role of the eldest child after an elder brother or sister died showed a similar intellectual advantage.

. 130 .
Why do twins develop different personalities?

If anything, the impact that genetics has on personality seems to be less strong at birth than later on in babyhood. A study of identical and nonidentical twins born in Kentucky found no similarity in terms of their irritability, resistance to soothing, activity level, or how responsive they were to sounds and objects during their first week of life, despite identical twins sharing the same DNA. So what else could account for the differences seen between twins? Although twins share the same uterus, they don't necessarily have the same experience while they're in there. Twins are often different sizes at birth, because the nutrients they receive aren't distributed equally. One twin may have a more difficult birth than the other one, and if there are complications, they may receive different treatment in the hospital. Even after they get home, they may be fed or attended to in different orders or by different parents. And if one twin starts to behave in a certain way—waking more frequently at night, for example—then its parents may start to treat it differently, giving it more hugs or having less patience when it cries.

Twins do seem to become more like each other toward the end of the first year, but they're still far from identical. As children age and have increasingly different experiences, their personalities diverge even further. But it's not just personality. You might assume that twins with identical DNA would be at the same risk of diseases such as diabetes, schizophrenia, or heart disease, but they're not. Neither do they tend to die from the same cause. Just why this should be is currently the source of intense research, but a likely explanation is that different experiences cause their genes to be more or less turned on or off through a process called epigenetics.

. 131 .
Do babies like some people better than others?

Some people love babies; others can't stand them. The funny thing is that babies may feel the same way about us. Given a choice between two faces—one attractive and one unattractive—a newborn baby will choose to fixate on the beautiful face. Alan Slater and his colleagues at the University of Exeter, UK, asked adults to rate a variety of female faces on attractiveness, then searched for pairs of photographs that were well matched for brightness and contrast but at opposite ends of the attractiveness spectrum.

These photos were then shown to babies ranging from one to seven days old, while a researcher stood out of sight and noted in which direction their eyes moved. Nearly all of the babies fixated on the more attractive face.

Slater suggests that faces we judge to be more attractive come closer to the prototype for a human face, which babies are hardwired to recognize (see 78: "What do newborns know?"). Previous research has shown that if you meld together lots of different faces to create a single one, the face you come up with is rated as extremely attractive by many.

But babies don't just judge books by their covers. Newborns also get upset if people's facial expressions suggest they're not responding to them. Experiments with babies as young as three hours old have shown that if their mother pulls a blank, expressionless face, the baby responds by decreasing eye contact and showing signs of distress. This suggests that babies are born with certain expectations regarding the rules of interpersonal communication. It might also explain why babies start to cry if someone glares at them.

By the age of six months, babies seem to have become pretty good judges of character. Karen Wynn and her colleagues at Yale University showed twelve babies a puppet show in which different toys with googly eyes climbed up a hill, either helping or hindering one another. For example, in one scenario, a yellow triangle helped a red circle climb the hill, and then a blue square aggressively pushed it back down.

After the show had finished, the babies were offered all the toys to see which one they preferred. All twelve six-month-olds picked the helpful character. The researchers got a similar result when the same experiment was done with ten-month-olds.

When two of the blocks moved up the hill together, the babies seemed unsure which one they preferred, possibly because they were unsure of the blocks' intentions.

This experiment suggests that babies may start to make judgments about social situations about a year earlier than previously assumed. By around eighteen months of age, toddlers will actively start trying to be helpful, picking up a broom and trying to sweep the kitchen floor, for example.

. 132 .
How much do babies remember?

What is your earliest memory? Probably it was sometime between the age of two and four, though you may be confused about the details and wonder if it really happened at all. That's how I feel about my first memory: being pushed up a hill in Canada, eating from a packet of Fruit Loops. According to my mother, we did visit Canada when I was about two and a half, and I probably did eat Fruit Loops, but whether this is an actual memory is hard to tell.

For a long time, scientists believed that babies had no memory at all—something they called "infantile amnesia." But that view has changed in recent years, as we learn more about the different types of memory that exist and when these begin to form.

It's quite true that if you ask adults to recall their earliest memory, most can't remember anything before the age of two or three. There's some evidence that emotionally charged events are the most memorable. One study that asked college students whether they could recall life-changing events that happened before they were five years old found that memories of being hospitalized or the birth of a sibling seemed to be particularly memorable, as details could be recalled from around the age of two, while the death of a family member or moving to a new home tended to be recalled if it happened after they were three.

This period of a child's development is marked by the emergence of two other skills that may help to explain why these "autobiographical memories" don't seem to stick from an earlier age. One is a sense of "self," as autobiographical memories are characterized by the fact that they usually place you as an individual at the center of them. The other is language. Several studies have suggested that possessing the language to describe events and objects might help us to remember them. For one thing, it may provide children with extra prompts for accessing memories. Language also provides opportunities for rehearsing and reviving memories through conversations with family and friends. It may help in the laying down of memories in the first place; many parents notice how two- or three-year-olds sometimes lie in bed and seem to chatter through the day's events to themselves.

The importance of language in summoning memories was shown through an experiment using something called "the magic shrinking machine." Two- to three-year-old children were asked to take a toy from a box and put it into the top of the machine. They then pulled a lever, and a miniature version of the same toy appeared from a chute at the bottom of the machine (there was an adult sitting behind the machine who was selecting the appropriate toy to release from the chute). The children's language ability was assessed when they first saw the machine and again when they were asked about it either six months or a year later. When the children were asked what they remembered about the machine and how it worked, they were incapable of describing things they didn't have the appropriate vocabulary for at the time of first seeing it, even if their language ability was now very good. They simply couldn't find the words to describe it, even if they possessed those words now. However, it was clear the children remembered the machine, as they could use photographs to explain how it worked.

. 133 .
Why don't we remember being babies?

Just because adults can't remember their early childhoods, this doesn't mean that babies don't remember what happened to them from one day to the next. It's clear that even fetuses have the ability to learn, which requires some degree of memory. For example, newborns seem to recognize pieces of music that were played to them and individual voices they heard before birth (see 36: "What do babies learn during their time in the womb?"). This is different than autobiographical memory, but it is memory nonetheless.

In general, the older a baby is, the longer it will hold on to memories. Some of the most famous experiments investigating memory in tiny babies were done by Carolyn Rovee-Collier, now at Rutgers University. She took babies as young as two months and attached one of their feet by a ribbon to the brightly colored mobile that hung above their crib. If the babies kicked their feet, the mobile would move, and if they kicked really hard, the figures would knock against each other, producing a clanking sound—a very exciting thing for a nine-week-old.

After playing this game for two nine-minute sessions, the babies were tested days later to see how long they would remember that they had to kick their feet in order to get the mobile to move. Two-month-old babies held on to this knowledge for just one to two days, but six-month-old babies could remember it for two weeks.

How many times they got to play the game made a big difference to how long they remembered it. If the two-month-olds were given three six-minute training sessions, for example, they could remember the game for two weeks.

One theory is that babies have no problem laying down memories; the problem is retrieving them. This could also explain why we adults struggle to access memories from our early years: Our view of the world has changed so much that the simple cues that once triggered memories—that enormous, looming chair, or the colorful buttons on our mother's sweater—are no longer present or no longer carry the same salience as they did when we were tiny babies.

In a later experiment, Rovee-Collier found that periodically reminding babies of the mobile game by simply showing them the mobile (but not actually attaching their foot to it) extended their memory of it. Three-month-olds given two nine-minute training sessions generally couldn't remember to kick their feet when they were tested two weeks later, but if they were shown the same mobile twenty-four hours before the test, they could. It's as if seeing the mobile enabled them to replay the game in their heads, so when they were tested twenty-four hours later, they knew exactly what to do.

But these kinds of experiments test only a baby's ability to remember skills or habits, which isn't the same as consciously remembering experiences such as a trip to the circus or the cake your grandmother baked for your first birthday. Obviously, this type of memory is difficult to assess in babies, because they can't tell us what they can remember, but Andrew Meltzoff of the University of Washington has found an indirect way of testing it.

He decided to show babies unexpected ways of using several new objects, such as a cup that collapses if you press down on it from above and a box that lights up when you touch it with your forehead. The question was whether babies would remember what to do with these objects if they'd watched an adult using them but never handled the objects themselves.

When he did this with fourteen-month-old babies, he found that when they were given the objects two to four months later, many of them immediately picked them up and imitated what they had seen the adults do with them. Similar studies have hinted that babies as young as nine months may have this ability to remember things without directly experiencing them first.

The memory tests aren't perfect, and they don't necessarily reflect real life, when babies may be exposed to objects or experiences repeatedly, or in different situations and contexts, but they suggest that babies have strong memories, even if they can't recall them when they grow up. It is unclear how modern technologies such as digital cameras and video might influence children's ability to remember things. When my daughter, Matilda, was around twenty months old, she became obsessed with watching a recording of some circus horses and their trainer, Yasmine Smart, whom we'd seen performing at Zippos Circus in London several weeks earlier. After visiting the circus, Matilda asked to watch the video almost every day. I'm fascinated to know whether she will retain the memory of that circus visit for many years to come—although I will have to ask her about other details of the circus besides the horses, to be sure she isn't just remembering the video.

134.
Does day care make babies sociable or stressed?

Should you decide to go back to work, choosing child care for your baby is likely to be one of the most stressful decisions you'll make. Newspaper headlines warning that babies who attend day care experience damaging levels of stress hormones only serve to make parental guilt worse, yet many of us have little option. On the other hand, there's the nagging feeling that playing with other children is likely to be good for a baby's social development, so maybe day care is a positive thing after all.

Cortisol is a hormone that is released during normal daily activity, but it is also released in large amounts in response to stress. Several studies have found that children attending full-day child care have higher levels of cortisol on the afternoons they attend child care compared to days when they are at home with their parents (a pattern also seen in adult executives working in high-stress jobs). For example, one study of toddlers aged eighteen months to three years old found that afternoon cortisol levels were one and a half times higher on the days the toddlers attended day care, even though the centers they attended scored highly on measures of child-care quality. But is stress an inevitable consequence of being separated from one's parents? To investigate, Andrea Dettling of the Swiss Federal Institute of Technology compared three- to four-year-olds who were placed in day care for around forty hours a week with those who spent similar amounts of time away from home with a care provider, and with those who received no external child care. It was a small study, with just twenty children in each group, but it did find that being separated from one's parents for the day isn't necessarily stressful in itself. Although children attending day care showed greater release of cortisol in the afternoon (as had been seen in previous studies), cortisol release among children being looked after by care provider depended on the amount of individual attention the child received from the carer. Those whose care provider gave them plenty of individual attention showed no difference in cortisol levels compared to when they stayed at home, while those who received lower-quality child care showed patterns similar to those children attending day care.

Even if day care does raise children's cortisol levels, that doesn't necessarily cause any long-term damage. One of the largest studies to address these issues is the Study of Early Child Care (SECC), funded by the U.S. National Institute of Child Health and Human Development. It has followed the development of more than twelve hundred children from birth through to middle childhood.

On the whole, it has found that children cared for exclusively by their mothers do not develop differently from those who are also cared for by others. Those who receive high-quality child care get some additional benefits, including slightly better cognitive function and language development across the first three years of life and greater school readiness at four and a half—although the effect is small compared to the influence that individual parents have on their children's development. This means that children whose parents don't have the time or inclination to interact with them may benefit from attending day care, but the benefit is likely to be small if they receive such stimulation at home. In terms of boosting young children's cognitive and language development, the most important aspect seems to be asking children questions, responding to their attempts to speak, and engaging them in other forms of communication, such as singing songs, reading books, and getting them to repeat numbers, shapes, or letters.

It's a similar picture when it comes to children's social and emotional development. The SECC study has found that quality of parenting has a far greater impact on this aspect of development than whether children are regularly cared for by someone else, or on the quality, quantity, or stability of the care. That's not to say that child care has no effect: Higher-quality care results in greater social competence, cooperation, and less problematic behavior at two and three years of age, compared to lower quality care.

It's also true that greater experience in groups with other children (regardless of whether they get this through attending day care or by going to toddler groups with their parents) makes young children slightly more cooperative and better at interacting with others as they get older. Other studies have hinted that children who attend day care are more accomplished at entertaining themselves, have greater self-confidence, and show less distress in new situations. The amount of time children spend in care also has an effect. Being in child care for thirty or more hours a week is associated with a small but statistically significant increase in behavioral problems.

Finally, it's worth noting that some children appear to be more affected by poor-quality child care and get more out of high-quality child care than others. In particular, babies who are fussy, difficult to soothe, and irritable tend to experience more behavioral problems when faced with low-quality child care but fewer behavioral problems than those with easy temperaments if they experience high-quality child care. These difficult babies may even be rated as more socially competent than children with easy temperaments, provided they receive sensitive and encouraging care from their minders.

So how can parents judge the quality of care that a nanny or day-care provider is offering? Generally speaking, higher levels of education and training among caregivers seem to be associated with better-quality care, as does having a low ratio of children to adults and a small overall group or class size. For babies aged six to eighteen months, the American Academy of Pediatrics recommends having no more than three babies to one adult and limiting overall group size to six babies. For eighteen- to twenty-four-month-olds, it suggests no more than four toddlers to one adult and limiting groups to eight.

Researchers in the SECC study have also concluded that high-quality child care hinges upon sensitive, encouraging, and frequent interactions between the caregiver and the child—something that may be harder to achieve within larger groups, or if a caregiver has too many children to look after.

In order to assess this, they recommend that parents look out for the following signs when choosing child care, all of which are markers of high-quality care:

- Is the caregiver generally in good spirits and encouraging when interacting with the child?
- Does the caregiver hug the child, pat the child on the back, or hold the child's hand? Does the caregiver offer comfort if the child is upset?
- Does the caregiver repeat the child's words, comment on what the child says or tries to say, and answer the child's questions?
- Does the caregiver encourage the child to talk/communicate by asking questions that the child can answer easily, such as yes-or-no questions, or asking about a family member or a toy?

- Does the caregiver respond to the child's positive actions with positive words, such as "You did it!" or "Well done!"? Does the minder encourage the child to say the alphabet out loud, count to ten, and name shapes or objects?
- Does the caregiver tell stories, describe objects or events, or sing songs?
- Does the caregiver encourage development by, for example, giving young babies tummy time to help neck and shoulder muscles grow stronger, helping older babies to walk or to finish puzzles, stack blocks, or zip zippers?
- Does the caregiver encourage the child to smile, laugh, and play with other children? Does the caregiver support sharing between the child and other children and provide examples of good behavior?
- Does the caregiver read books and stories to the child? Does the caregiver let the child touch the book and turn the pages?
- Does the caregiver ensure that she is positive, not negative, in interactions with the child, even when the child is misbehaving? Does the caregiver make it a point to interact with the child and not ignore him or her?

. 135 .
Are babies born in summer any different from winter babies?

Although your baby may not show the enthusiasm of a Leo or the precision of a Virgo, consider this: If he was born in the U.S. during August, he's nearly twice as likely to become a major league baseball player as a baby born a month earlier.

It's the same story in the UK, where babies born between September and December are twice as likely to become professional soccer players compared to those born in the summer months; unfortunately, they're also slightly more likely to suffer panic attacks and, if they're male, to become alcoholic when they get older. Meanwhile, if you're ambitious for your child to become a doctor, you might aim for an April to June birthday (at least if you live in the northern hemisphere).

There is also some evidence that a baby's season of birth can influence its health. For example, babies born in the northern hemisphere between December and April are more likely to develop schizophrenia or bipolar disorder than those born at other times of the year, while babies born between April and June are at greater risk of developing anorexia.

The effect of your birth month on all of these things is small, of course, but it is too great to be dismissed as chance. The risk of schizophrenia (which is among the best studied of these season-linked disorders) for babies born in the northern hemisphere during February, March, and April is around 5 to 10 percent higher than for babies born at other times of the year. This is similar to the increased risk associated with having a parent or sibling with the disorder. Scientists have proposed some mechanisms by which these trends might come about. In the case of sports, something called the relative age effect has been used to explain why babies born at certain times of the year are more likely to become professional players. For example, the cutoff date for almost all nonschool baseball leagues is July 31, meaning that kids born in August tend to be more physically mature and have had more time to practice their pitching than those born eleven months later.

Different factors are likely to be at work when it comes to health. Some studies have suggested that the increased risk of schizophrenia among babies born in the springtime is the result of the mother being exposed to viruses such as influenza during a critical period of pregnancy. More recently, scientists have proposed that vitamin D deficiency caused by low levels of sunlight during pregnancy may be to blame, or that varying levels of brain chemicals such as serotonin or dopamine at different times of the year might play a role.

In some countries, a baby's season of birth can influence physical development. The city of Denver nestles in the heart of the Rocky Mountains, so it experiences some pretty harsh winters. A study of 425 babies living there found that those born in summer and autumn started crawling around three weeks later on average than babies born in winter. Babies typically start to crawl between six and eight months—the height of winter for an American baby born during the summer months. Fewer daylight hours, not to mention the snow and biting cold, mean that such babies will probably spend more time bundled up in a cozy stroller rather than getting out and practicing their fledgling crawling skills. By contrast, babies born in winter are learning to crawl at precisely the time when they are most likely to have the space and motivation to explore their surroundings: summer. Other studies have confirmed that physically active babies who start to practice crawling or stepping actions earlier also tend to be the first ones to get on the move—usually much to the consternation of their frazzled mothers.

. 136 .
Does being born at the start of the school year give you an academic advantage?

It might, although the effect diminishes with age. Numerous studies have found that children born at the start of the academic year tend to score higher on tests than children who are the youngest in their year group. A recent analysis of birth dates among the CEOs of S&P 500 companies similarly found far fewer June- and July-borns among their ranks, possibly because high school leaders tend to be kids who are flourishing academically. As the admission cutoff dates for U.S. schools typically falls between September 1 and January 1, children born in June and July tend to be the youngest in their class and may struggle academically.

One of the largest studies to look at this issue was conducted in England, where the academic year also starts in September. By the age of seven, August-born children are two to three times as likely to be rated as "below average" by their teachers in reading, writing, and arithmetic. For example, 14 percent of September-born children were rated "below average" on their reading ability, compared to 30 percent of August-born children. The gap seems to narrow as children age, suggesting that August-borns do make up some of the lost ground. Overall, around half of children in England attain five GCSEs (exams taken at sixteen) at grades A to C, including English and math. However, if you compare children born in August with those born the previous September, girls are 5.5 percent less likely to hit this target, while boys are 6.1 percent less likely to do so. The same researchers found that

August-born teenagers are 20 percent less likely to get into top universities such as Oxford or Cambridge than their September-born counterparts. Despite all this, the researchers found no difference in children's sense of self-worth, their enjoyment of school, or their expectations of and aspirations for further and higher education.

The jury is still out on what's to blame for the disparity or what to do about it. One possibility is that August-born children simply aren't ready to start school at the age of four and so don't benefit from formal education during this time; another is that it's down to making children sit the tests on the same day, regardless of age.

Another problem is that such studies don't take into account the abilities of individual children. For example, we don't know if August-born children with high IQs would be similarly affected by their date of birth or if this would buffer them from the effect. Neither is it clear whether children who attend nursery school or whose parents spend a lot of time reading to them before they start school are similarly disadvantaged.

What is clear is that there are plenty of August-born geniuses to testify that there are always exceptions to the rule.

Language

. 137 .
When will my baby understand what I'm saying?

Most children begin to utter their first words around their first birthday. Until very recently, babies younger than ten to twelve months were referred to as "pre-linguistic": Although they could recognize the common vowel and consonant sounds produced by those around them, they couldn't understand the meaning of actual words. A popular theory was that babies couldn't grasp language until they started viewing other people as individuals with their own motivations, which generally begins around nine to ten months. Before this, they didn't understand enough about people's intentions to associate these sounds with actual things or actions.

New research is starting to challenge that view. Elika Bergelson and Daniel Swingley at the University of Pennsylvania tested the ability of six- and nine-month-olds to link words for food and body parts to the appropriate pictures by prompting them to "look at the apple" and then tracking their eye movements. They found that babies as young as six months were capable of identifying the correct object—including when it formed part of a picture containing several objects, such as a kitchen table with an apple, a cookie, yogurt, and a bottle on it.

The message we can take from this is that even young babies may understand some of what is said to them, so it makes sense to talk to them as much as possible. Research on older babies has shown that engaging babies in conversation is a far more effective way of teaching language than leaving them to absorb it passively, even if they don't answer back yet.

. 138 .
Why do babies say "Dada" before "Mama"?

Learning to speak requires the coordination of more than seventy different muscles and body parts and is one of the most complicated physical actions we humans perform. Perhaps it's no wonder that fully mastering language takes children around five years.

At around seven or eight months of age, babies start to babble. Barbara L. Davis at the University of Texas in Austin travels the world trying to capture some of these first utterances and make sense of them. Using tiny microphones attached to babies' bibs, she has recorded babble from as far afield as China, Ecuador, and Romania. She's also heard American, French, Dutch, and Berber babies babble. "What we've found is that children are extremely alike during this babbling period," she says.

Sounds such as "b," "d," "m," and "g" combined with "ah" seem to be the easiest to make, so that's where babies start. "You open and close your lips and you get 'ba ba ba,' " says Davis. Babies can't control their tongues very well, so they cannot articulate other sounds, but they can move them forward and backward. "If you put your tongue at the front of the mouth, you get 'da da da,' and if you move it to the back, you get 'ga ga ga,' " says Davis.

At this stage, babies are not necessarily trying to communicate; they are simply producing rhythmic sounds that will provide the foundation of later language. Although many parents assume that "Mama" and "Dada" are among a baby's first words because these are the people who are most important to them, baby babble isn't thought to start taking on meaning until around ten months to a year. So if your baby says "Dada" before "Mama," it doesn't mean he or she likes Daddy best.

Many babies do tend to say "da" before "ma." "Early speech sounds tend to be produced by moving the lips, jaw, and soft palate simultaneously," says Jordan Green at the University of Nebraska in Lincoln. This is how we make "ba" and "da" sounds, whereas "ma" requires us to move the lips and jaw but relax the soft palate so the sound enters the nasal cavity.

Adults use "da" and "ba" more frequently than they use "ma" and "na," and babies seem to have figured this out. " 'Da' is the most common sound across the world's languages," says Davis. "Probably the reason they are saying 'Dada' sooner than 'Mama' is because they are making more of these oral sounds."

It could even be that the very reason these words exist is because, throughout history, parents have seized babies' first utterances and used them to label themselves. Indeed, the baby words for "mother" and "father" are remarkably similar across languages. Father is "dada," "papa," "baba," and "abba" in English, French, Chinese/Persian, and Aramaic, respectively; "mama" is the same across English, Chinese, and Swahili, and is "haha" in Japanese. There are exceptions, such as "chichi," which is Japanese for "father," but these seem to be in the minority.

Some of the hardest sounds to make are "r," "l," "ph," "ch," and "sh," so these tend to be some of the last sounds that children master. This explains why many toddlers say adorable-sounding words like "babbit" instead of "rabbit."

139.
When does baby babble take on meaning?

Although babies start babbling at around seven months, most language experts believe it takes at least a few more months before baby babble morphs into something more meaningful. On average, babies say their first words at around the age of one, although there is enormous variability in when babies start to speak. Some babies don't babble at all and move straight into speech. "There are children who are relatively more or less voluble, but it's certainly something to pay attention to if there's none of it, or if they continue making 'buuuuuuuh' or 'muuuuuuuh' sounds that aren't very rhythmic and syllable-like," says Barbara Davis.

Recent studies have found that babbling may be more than simple mouth movements, however. You may never have noticed it, but when people talk, the right side of their mouth opens a tiny bit wider than the left. This is because the left side of the brain (which controls the right side of the face) plays a greater role in producing language. To investigate whether babbling might be a first shot at language, Laura-Ann Petitto and her colleagues filmed ten babies between five and twelve months while they were babbling, making other noises, or smiling. She then slowed down the tapes and asked people who knew nothing about the study to rate which side of the babies' mouths opened more.

Sure enough, when the babies were babbling, they showed the same pattern of mouth opening as adults, suggesting that the language areas of their brains were being used. Smiling had the opposite effect, which may be because the right side of the brain is more involved in processing emotions.

When they do appear, first words often contain many of the same sounds as early babbling, which makes it even more difficult to detect precisely when babbling ends and words begin. Parents are generally better than strangers at spotting the transition, because they spend every day with their babies and can spot patterns such as saying "ba" every time the baby gets into the bath.

Although words for people and objects are relatively easy to identify, studies suggest that several nonobject words such as "gone," "there," "uh-oh," and "more" are also among a baby's early vocal repertoire. During the 1980s, Alison Gopnik of the University of California in Berkeley recorded one-year-olds going about their daily business in order to find out what words they were using and how they were using them. In her book *The Scientist in the Crib,* she describes how an eighteen-month-old named Henry repeatedly used the word "gone" to describe the many and varied ways in which objects disappear from view, rather than meaning that something is finished, like dinner.

Similarly, babies often use "oh dear" or "uh-oh" to describe failures, and "there" to indicate success. They extend naming words to other people or objects with similar characteristics, so male friends and the postman become "Dada," and the definition of "moon" is extended to include all manner of lamps, oranges, and fingernail clippings. My daughter has taken to using "bumpy head" whenever she is upset or frustrated. Clearly, she associates crying with a time when she bumped her head and feels that this is the most appropriate way to describe her emotions.

. 140 .
Do babies communicate without language?

Babies clearly understand that crying elicits attention, but they soon develop other means of communication as well. Stick your tongue out at one-month-olds, and often they'll stick theirs out back. Talk to young babies, and you may notice them stop moving and responding with a volley of wriggles, coos, and smiles. All this suggests that even young babies understand the fundamentals of communication and get better at it with every passing day.

Babies love having their own actions mimicked. One study found that three-and-a-half-month-old babies cooed and smiled more frequently when moms imitated their sounds and expressions compared to when they responded with different sounds and actions.

As babies progress from cooing to babbling, they begin to realize that they can use these sounds to get adults to interact with them—a bit like starting a conversation. In a recent study, Michael Goldstein and his colleagues at Cornell University studied how five-month-olds reacted when an adult they had been playing with suddenly assumed an expressionless face and started ignoring them. Babies hate this. If you do it to a younger infant, she will invariably look away and start to cry. But the five-month-olds reacted differently. Rather than crying, they increased their coos and squeals, apparently trying to engage the adult in conversation. When they got nothing back, they eventually stopped trying and just looked sad.

At around the age of one, babies start pointing. The traditional view is that they do this only to get things they want, but more recent studies suggest that one-year-olds also point in order to be helpful. This is surprising, because helpfulness implies an understanding that other people have minds of their own and don't necessarily know everything you do—a complex social skill that wasn't thought to develop until later.

Ulf Liszkowski and colleagues at the Max Planck Institute for Psycholinguistics in Nijmegen, the Netherlands, sat one-year-olds at a table and did craft projects with them. For example, they took an ink stamp and used it to print on a piece of paper, then took a roll of tape and used it to stick the edges of a piece of cloth together. Then they did it again, this time deliberately knocking the roll of tape off the edge of the table, down a chute, and on the floor. When it came to the moment when the tape was needed, the adult began to hunt for it. In nearly every case, the one-year-olds pointed to the dropped tape in order to help them find it.

This suggests that one-year-olds understand others' ignorance and want to help them. Even though they can't yet say "You've dropped something," they can tell them by using the newly acquired pointing skill.

. 141 .
Do more physical babies develop language faster than sedentary babies?

Any parent will tell you that babies are different. Some are more sociable, others more active, but it seems the very act of starting to move about marks a change in the way they interact with other people. Several studies have shown that once babies start to crawl, they show both more anger and affection toward their parents, more sensitivity to their comings and goings, and more attention to what's going on around them. What's more, it seems to be the act of movement that triggers these changes, rather than the other way around. If you put a baby who can't yet crawl into a walker, it behaves very differently than when it is left lying on a play mat. When they can't move, babies are less sociable and mostly focus on items on the floor. But put them in a walker and they behave just like mobile infants of the same age, engaging with adults in the room and looking at things on the walls. It seems that this new perspective on the world somehow stimulates them to become more sociable. Possibly, it's that they can see more once they've started crawling or are upright.

The transition to walking also seems to trigger a change in babies' social behavior. Melissa Clearfield of Whitman College in Walla Walla, Washington, compared nine- to twelve-month-olds who could walk with babies of the same age who were still crawling but could stand upright and move about the room in a walker. She found that babies who could walk independently spent more time interacting with toys and their mothers. They also made more attempts to babble or speak, and more gestures, such as pointing or waving at a toy while looking at their mothers. Importantly, the babies in the walker had their hands free and could have done the same things, but they didn't. It seems the transition to independent walking itself changes how babies interact with others.

. 142 .
Why do women speak to babies in a silly voice?

"Coochy-coo." "Want Mama to play with that?" Let's face it, we've all caught ourselves speaking like idiots when a baby is around, but there's a genuine reason for doing it: Babies like it. Given a choice between listening to a mom talking to a baby and the same mom talking to another adult, babies will choose the baby talk. It even has a proper name: motherese.

Parents across the world show a common pattern when talking to babies. They raise the pitch of their voice, speak more slowly, elongate the vowels, and exaggerate changes in intonation, giving their speech an almost musical quality. Sentences are shortened, and subtle variations of the same sentence are often repeated.

What's more, it seems that this unconscious shift to motherese may help babies to learn language. Previous studies have shown that English, Swedish, Chinese, and Russian mothers unconsciously tailor their motherese to make the vowels of their language particularly resonant, with phrases such as "Oooooh, you're so cuuute, with those biiig bluuue eeeyes." More recently, Jae Young Song and his colleagues at Brown University tested nineteen-month-olds and found that this elongation of vowel sounds significantly enhanced the ability to recognize words.

It's not only our voices; recent research has shown that we change our behavior, too. Mothers were recorded showing a series of toys to adults and babies, including a snake made up of a string of colored wooden beads and a clear plastic hamster ball that contained a smaller colored ball. Compared to when they showed adults how these toys worked, the women were more interactive, enthusiastic, and repetitive when they demonstrated them to babies. What's more, given a choice between watching the adult-directed demonstration and the baby-directed one, babies were far more interested in the one that moms had instinctively tailored to babies.

Dads also seem to change their physical behavior when they interact with babies, but in a slightly different way. When dads demonstrated the same toys to infants, they were slightly less enthusiastic than the mothers, but they seemed to get closer to the babies and allow them more opportunities to touch and explore how the toy worked. This desire to demonstrate the intricacies of how things work has been seen in studies that have looked at how fatherly behavior is influenced by hormones such as prolactin (see 32: "Do men change when they become dads?"), so I wonder if it's a more general difference between men and women.

Such changes in physical behavior might be important in capturing babies' attention, as well as teaching them about human motivation and how to explore, test, and understand the things they come across in everyday life.

. 143 .
When do babies start learning language?

Babies are born with the ability to absorb any language, but even before birth, they are beginning to sift through the various sounds and rhythms they hear and trying to make sense of them. Four-day-old babies can distinguish the language they've heard in the womb from other languages (see 78: "What do newborns know?"), although it may take up to a year for them to utter their first word.

Even though babies start categorizing sounds and rhythms from birth, for around nine months, their brains remain "international" in the sense that they can discriminate all 150 speech sounds that occur across human languages. Think of adult Japanese speakers, who struggle to differentiate between the "r" and "l" sounds of English, or English speakers, who often fail to perceive the difference between "p" and "b" in Spanish and French. None of this is a problem for a young baby, who can detect these differences regardless of who is talking to them.

When Patricia Kuhl of the University of Washington set out to test this language ability of babies across continents, she found a curious pattern: At some point during the second half of the first year, it switches off. Japanese babies who were perfectly capable of perceiving the difference between "r" and "l" at seven months (as measured by their tendency to turn their head toward the loudspeaker when the sounds changed) were incapable of discriminating between them by eleven months of age. It's as if the brain gradually starts to filter out sounds that are irrelevant in everyday life.

Whether it's possible to regain this universal sound perception is a matter of debate. For a long time the answer was thought to be no, but Kuhl's recent studies have hinted that babies' ears can be kept open to other languages, given the right stimulation. When she exposed nine-month-old American babies to twelve twenty-five-minute language sessions over the course of a month, in which a Mandarin speaker read from children's books and played with puppets, a train, and stacks of rings, she found that these babies retained the ability to perceive Mandarin sounds when other American babies of the same age lost it. Importantly, this happened only if the babies were exposed to Mandarin speakers in the flesh—it didn't work if they were played a DVD in Mandarin. It's unclear how long the effect lasts. In Kuhl's study, the babies retained their ear for Mandarin for at least two weeks after last hearing it; unfortunately, they weren't tested again after that.

. 144 .
When is the best time to introduce a second language?

A key question that has troubled parents and linguists alike is whether children should master one language before attempting to tackle a second one. The fear has been that they may confuse the two languages or fall behind their peers who are learning one. Laura-Ann Petitto of Gallaudet University has spent her career investigating how babies acquire language. She even spent some time trying to teach a chimpanzee to learn sign language.

Her research suggests that the fear is unfounded. She tested children who had been exposed to both French and English or French and sign language from birth and compared the age at which they reached language milestones, such as speaking their first word or stringing words together in a sentence, with children learning just one language. The bilingual children achieved these milestones at the same age, despite having spent only half as much time being exposed to either language.

"Considerable research now suggests that learning two languages is as natural as learning one and that, given the right learning environment, most children can acquire two languages simultaneously at the same rate and in the same way as monolingual children," says Fred Genesee, a bilingualism expert at McGill University.

Another myth is the "one parent, one language" rule, or bilingual parents sticking to a single language in the company of their child to avoid confusing it. "There's absolutely no evidence that that's true," says Genesee. "However, it's not a bad strategy to use because it guarantees at least a minimum exposure to the minority language."

If a baby lives in a house where more than one language is spoken, or if its mother speaks a different language than that of the community she's living in, the baby probably starts learning aspects of those languages even before birth. "Starting at that point makes sense for children for whom being bilingual is really important, or who are likely to keep on being exposed to a language once they're born," says Genesee. "There's a lot of evidence suggesting that the first year or two establishes some critical foundations for language learning."

What about monolingual parents who would like their child to be able to speak more than one language? Although there's no evidence that exposing babies to more than one language is harmful, it could be a waste of time, because they're unlikely to experience enough of it to learn very much. Research suggests that children need to spend between 30 and 50 percent of their day hearing a particular language in order to become as good at it as a monolingual child. This suggests that my mother-in-law's attempts to teach our children French when she sees them every six weeks are unlikely to result in any degree of fluency, although it may help tune their ears to French, which could have benefits if they choose to study it when they're older.

In order to become proficient in a language, young children typically need two to three years of exposure. Immersing a young child in a foreign language for a few months would probably be enough to give him a good grounding in it, particularly if he is interacting with other children, but Genesee cautions against trying to bombard children with too many languages, as could happen if parents are regularly moving from country to country. "What could be detrimental is if children are exposed to more than two or three languages and that exposure is fragmented and not extensive enough," he says.

The Next One

. 145 .
Are women more fertile after having a baby?

Parenting chat rooms are filled with anecdotal reports that women are super-fertile after having had a baby. Similar rumors abound about miscarriage, with many women claiming that their doctor has told them they're more likely to conceive after a miscarriage because their hormone levels are more favorable.

Surprisingly, there's no research to either support or refute reports of extreme fertility in women who have already conceived a child. While some women appear to have been told that high progesterone levels following a miscarriage or pregnancy make them more likely to conceive, there is no published evidence to suggest that this is true.

Progesterone is a hormone produced in large amounts during pregnancy, as well as at certain times during the menstrual cycle. It causes the lining of the uterus—the endometrium—to thicken, which theoretically could help a fertilized egg to implant. Indeed, some researchers are experimenting with progesterone to improve success rates during fertility treatment. However, "it is not likely that progesterone remains at a high enough concentration to have an effect the month after a miscarriage," says Anneli Stavreus Evers, a reproductive endocrinologist at Uppsala University Hospital in Sweden, who is leading some of these efforts. After a miscarriage, the lining of the uterus will be shed, as with a normal period, and after that, the lining should develop in the same way as during a normal menstrual cycle. What's more, high progesterone at the wrong time of the menstrual cycle might actually impede implantation.

Another possibility is that previous pregnancies might stimulate improvements in medical conditions associated with reduced fertility. For example, changes in hormone levels during pregnancy could cause the regression of endometriosis, a common condition in which cells from the lining of the uterus grow elsewhere, while the growing uterus could cause the dissolving of scar tissue within the uterus (caused by previous infections or surgery), says Caleb Kallen, a reproductive endocrinologist and fertility expert at Emory University School of Medicine. Some women who had infrequent periods before pregnancy find that their periods become more regular after having a baby. However, such fertility changes have never been systematically studied and are unlikely to affect more than a small minority of women. "I am not aware of any genuine fertility or hormonal benefits stemming from delivering a baby," says Kallen.

. 146 .
Am I likely to become pregnant when breast-feeding?

Your chances of getting pregnant are greatly reduced, but it's no guarantee. Several studies have shown that if a woman suckles her baby more than five times a day for at least an hour in total, then she is highly unlikely to get pregnant (assuming the baby is latching on properly and feeding). The odds increase slightly after about six months, when babies start eating solids, but women who continue to breast-feed and aren't having periods are still unlikely to conceive.

The main trigger for this temporary infertility is the physical act of sucking the nipple. The maturation of eggs in the ovaries is controlled by a delicate balance of hormones that act as a kind of clock. The brain usually produces regular pulses of a hormone called gonadotropin-releasing hormone (GnRH), which in turn causes the release of another hormone called luteinizing hormone (LH), and this is what causes eggs to mature. The timing of these pulses is essential: GnRH needs to be released around once an hour for the right dose of LH to be secreted. Suckling slows the timing of these pulses, and if it slows too much, the result is temporary infertility.

When women stop breast-feeding, the pulses of GnRH begin to speed up again, but the rate at which this happens isn't the same for everybody. Some women who stop breast-feeding suddenly will become pregnant without even having a period; for others, it takes time for the balance of these hormones to reestablish themselves. This is especially true if you stop breast-feeding during the first six months after having a baby. "Even in the absence of breast-feeding, the return of ovulation is delayed," says Ronald Gray of Johns Hopkins Bloomberg School of Public Health in Baltimore. Indeed, many of the first bleeds that women experience after having a baby don't involve the release of an egg.

To confuse things further, mothers who slowly cut down their breast-feeding may find that their periods resume, even though they aren't ovulating and remain temporarily infertile. This is because pulses of GnRH have increased enough for the ovaries to start producing hormones that cause the uterine lining to thicken, but the signal isn't strong enough to mature an egg. When no egg is released, these hormone levels fall and women experience a period, even though they haven't ovulated.

. 147 .
I had no problem getting pregnant last time, so why am I struggling to conceive now?

While some women get pregnant on the first attempt, others struggle to conceive a second child, despite having found it relatively easy to get pregnant the first time around. Such "secondary infertility" can be tough to bear, particularly if well-meaning friends and relatives are constantly asking when the first child is going to get a sibling.

According to RESOLVE: The National Infertility Association, approximately 30 percent of couples seeking help with infertility already have at least one child, and secondary infertility seems to be on the rise—up from around 1.8 million cases per year in the U.S. in 1995 to nearly 3 million in 2006. Despite this, there is little research into the causes of secondary infertility, as it is assumed that the causes are the same as those affecting couples who have never had a baby.

There are, however, some known mechanisms by which having a child might reduce subsequent fertility. The most obvious is breast-feeding, which vastly reduces a woman's chances of ovulating and becoming pregnant, at least during the first six months. Even if your periods have resumed, this doesn't mean that you are ovulating, as it can take time for the hormones that drive egg production in the ovaries to rebalance (see 146: "Am I likely to become pregnant when breast-feeding?").

Ovulation might also be delayed if the body isn't getting enough energy to supply its needs. Claudia Valeggia at the University of Pennsylvania recently measured hormone levels in seventy breast-feeding mothers in Toba, Argentina, and found that the average length of infertility after giving birth was 4.3 months. Closer analysis revealed that levels of insulin, which is produced in response to food, were low during the early months. This could be a sign that the women's energy supplies were in the red, possibly because the body needs a lot of energy to rebuild itself after pregnancy and birth.

Insulin helps the ovaries to produce reproductive hormones such as estrogen and progesterone, so its availability may influence when women become fertile again. Shortly before the Toba women resumed ovulation, they experienced a surge of insulin and tended to gain a few pounds in weight. "Energy balance has a deep influence on the reproductive axis of women of all ages, so if you are trying to lose those 'baby kilos' after your pregnancy, that may influence your chances of conceiving again," says Valeggia. Carrying too many extra pounds may interfere with how your body responds to insulin, while the stress of trying to juggle a career while running around after a toddler may dent your fertility still further.

In a minority of women, pregnancy can affect the function of the thyroid gland, resulting in something called postpartum thyroiditis. Around 7 percent of women are estimated to develop this condition within the first year of giving birth; common symptoms include hair loss, tiredness, and depression. While all of these may be symptoms of new motherhood, thyroid function can affect your fertility, so it may be another thing to get checked out.

Some doctors believe that those suffering from secondary infertility may have always had an underlying problem, such as polycystic ovaries, and they simply got lucky the first time around. Fibroids also have a tendency to grow during pregnancy, so if they were already present, they could be having a greater impact on fertility.

Possibly the main culprit of secondary infertility is aging. There is a sharp decline in fertility after the age of thirty-five, so it can take longer to become pregnant. "That said, prior fertility success means that, at least historically, everything worked at least once. So there must have been an open tube, a functional uterus, an egg and a sperm," says Kallen.

If you are over the age of thirty-five and have been trying to conceive for longer than six months, you should seek medical advice. Tests can be done to determine whether you are ovulating and if your levels of thyroid hormones and insulin are normal. If you are under thirty-five, the current advice is to wait a year before seeking help. Disconcerting as secondary infertility may be, it is quite normal to take a year or two to conceive, regardless of how quickly you got pregnant the first time around.

. 148 .
Why do some women seem to give birth only to boys?

On January 17, 1995, an earthquake measuring 6.8 on the Richter scale hit Kobe in Japan, killing around 6,434 people, injuring many more, and leaving thousands homeless. Nine months later, the first babies who would have been conceived during that traumatic time were born. Whereas around 51.6 percent of babies born in Japan normally are male, in the Kobe area, this fell to 50.1 percent in the aftermath of the earthquake. Similar declines in male births have been seen following other disasters, including the collapse of the Twin Towers on 9/11, while an increase in male births was observed after World War I and World War II.

The received wisdom is that we all have an equal chance of having a son or daughter—that it's like flipping a coin, heads or tails—and families with "runs" of boys or girls are the product of coincidence. In fact, the coin is already weighted slightly in favor of boys, with approximately 106 boys born for every 100 girls worldwide (although this figure has fluctuated over the last century). No one really understands why (and the numbers eventually balance out, as males are more likely to die during childhood or before they have children), but we do know of several environmental factors that seem to influence the gender of children.

As a general rule, men produce approximately 50 percent "male" and 50 percent "female" sperm, but exposure to radiation or high levels of hormone-disrupting chemicals such as phthalates (which are added to plastics) seems to tip the balance in favor of "female" sperm carrying an X-chromosome. For example, twice as many girls as boys are being born in a Canadian First Nations tribe called the Aamjiwnaang, which lives next door to the Sarnia-Lambton Chemical Valley complex in Ontario. High levels of hexachlorobenzene (HCB) have been found in the local soil, while it is thought that phthalates are also being emitted from the complex, prompting some to speculate that these are skewing the sex ratio. Meanwhile, men working at the Sellafield nuclear plant in Cumbria, UK, are up to 40 percent more likely to have boys than girls, suggesting that small doses of radiation may have an effect on the sex ratio.

Exposure to high levels of chemicals and radiation is admittedly rare, but it does suggest that the possibility to skew sex ratios exists. More prosaically, recent research suggests that women working in high-stress jobs are more likely to give birth to daughters than sons. However, the effect was small: 54 percent of women in low-stress jobs had sons, compared with 47 percent of women in high-stress jobs. It also seemed to be influenced by how much money the father made, with high-salary dads slightly more likely to have sons.

Other studies have also found that male managers have more sons than their employees, as do men working in typically male occupations such as engineering. There are certain diseases that seem to cause women to produce more sons, such as polycystic ovarian syndrome and multiple sclerosis.

How could all of this be? From an evolutionary perspective, it makes more sense to have boys when times are good—they take slightly more energy to grow and prosper, but when they do, they have the potential to generate far more grandchildren than do daughters (at least they did in our ancestors' times) and so ensure the propagation of our genes. In lean times, daughters are a better guarantee of producing at least a couple of grandchildren, since men are less picky about a mate (or so the theory goes).

Times of extreme stress may prompt the release of hormones that tell the body that lean times are ahead, either killing off male sperm or making male embryos (which tend to be slightly more fragile) less likely to survive. Similar hormonal factors may be at work in the more everyday cases of occupation-related imbalances in the sex ratio.

It's possible that some men or women are inherently more likely to have boys than girls, although precisely why remains a mystery. In a study of 1,403,021 children born to 700,030 couples in Denmark, approximately 51.2 percent of first births were male. As couples went on to have more children, an interesting pattern began to emerge. Women who had boys in their first and second births seemed to keep on having boys. In couples who already had three boys, the chances of having a fourth boy were 52.4 percent, and this rose to 54.2 percent for a fifth child. No such pattern was seen in couples with girls. So it seems that once you start down the path of having boys, you're statistically more likely to keep having them.

A similar mechanism may lie behind the finding that men with lots of brothers are more likely to have sons, while those with many sisters tend to have daughters. Corry Gellatly at Newcastle University uncovered this trend after analyzing 927 family trees containing information on 556,387 people from Europe and North America stretching back to the year 1600. Once again, it seems to be only men who are affected by this, so if a woman has lots of sisters, it is irrelevant. Gellatly proposes that some as yet undiscovered gene can influence the proportion of X- and Y-bearing sperm, which would mean that the assumption that all men have equal numbers of X- and Y-carrying sperm is untrue. Age and beauty also enter into the equation. Several studies have found that the older you get, the less likely you are to have a son. One recent study found that 53 percent of teenage parents have sons, while among parents over forty, the proportion is just 35 percent. Satoshi Kanazawa of the London School of Economics reached this conclusion after analyzing data from the UK National Child Development study, which followed a population of 17,419 British-born children through their lives. Here, the effect seemed particularly pronounced among older mothers. Kanazawa calculates that for every year a woman ages, the odds of her first child being a boy decrease by 1.2 percent. Egg quality is an obvious suspect: Perhaps more fragile male fetuses are less able to survive with minor mutations in their DNA than females are.

Whatever the mechanism, Kanazawa believes there is a good evolutionary explanation for older parents having daughters rather than sons. Once conceived, there is little that parents can do to increase their daughters' future reproductive success beyond keeping them alive and healthy. Sons, on the other hand, traditionally needed more investment from their parents in order to make sure they inherited the family's status and resources. If a son's parents died before he reached maturity, he was unlikely to be powerful enough to defend the family's wealth and resources. And although an orphaned girl was also in a perilous predicament, she could find a husband to take care of her. (We're talking in evolutionary terms, not about modern-day society.) It therefore makes sense for older parents to have girls, Kanazawa says.

A friend of mine with two teenage daughters provided an alternative explanation: "Mothers need all the age and experience they can get to handle teenage girls, so best to have them as late as possible," she says. In addition, Kanazawa found that beautiful parents were statistically more likely to have daughters than unattractive parents. When children in the study were seven, their teachers were asked to rate them as "attractive," "unattractive," "scruffy and dirty," "underfed," or "abnormal features." When those children grew up, the proportion of sons among those rated attractive was 50 percent, compared to 52 percent among those who fell into the other physical categories.

Again, Kanazawa has an evolutionary explanation. Although physical attractiveness is important for both sexes, it is especially important for women. Men prefer to mate with attractive women regardless of whether it's a one-night stand or a long-term partnership, while other traits such as wealth and status may be more important for women seeking a long-term partner.

It's important to bear in mind that, with all these studies, the effect on the sex ratio is small, which means that many ugly, young, chilled-out wives of business executives will give birth to daughters, and many stressed, aging supermodels will have sons. But it's food for thought. The more people look into it, the less certain is the assumption that gender is a pure matter of chance.

. 149 .
Is there anything I can do to influence the gender of my baby?

The only way to guarantee the gender of your baby is to undergo clinical sex selection (which is illegal in most countries), which involves IVF. But there are several "natural" methods that may tip the balance slightly in your favor.

All babies carry two sex chromosomes (one from the mother and one from the father), which dictate their gender. Male babies carry an X and a Y chromosome, while female babies carry two X chromosomes. Since all eggs carry an X chromosome, it's the father's sperm that determines the sex of the baby. Men usually produce similar numbers of sperm bearing X and Y chromosomes, so it's largely potluck whether you end up with a baby boy or girl.

That's not to say that external factors don't have any influence. The most famous method for influencing your baby's gender is the Shettles Method, based on the premise that the X chromosome is larger than the Y chromosome, so it weighs slightly more and may slow "female" sperm. For this reason, couples wanting boys are told to have sex as close to the moment of ovulation as possible in the hope that male sperm will beat female sperm to the egg. Female sperm are supposedly more robust, which means that they can survive for longer in the harsh environment of the reproductive tract. For this reason, Shettles advises couples wanting a girl to have sex two to three days before ovulation and to aim for shallower penetration to increase the amount of time the sperm spend in the acidic environment of the vagina.

Several studies have set out to test the Shettles Method, but none has proved conclusively that it works. A key problem is that couples trying to conceive rarely have sex only once around the time of ovulation, and it's tricky to pinpoint the exact moment of ovulation. At most, you might increase your chances of having the boy or girl you want by a couple of percent, but that's nowhere near a guarantee. Plus, if you restrict the days on which you have

sex, you're less likely to get pregnant in the first place. Another common belief is that a woman's diet before pregnancy can influence the sex of a baby.
A survey of 740 pregnant women found that 56 percent of women who ate a
high-energy diet before getting pregnant had boys, compared with 46 percent
who ate low-calorie diets.

One possibility is that women who eat more have higher blood-sugar levels, and this favors the survival of male embryos, something that has been
noticed when embryos are grown in IVF clinics. Women who gain weight
between their first and second pregnancies seem more prone to having boys
the second time around, whereas women with anorexia nervosa seem more
likely to have girls.

This makes sense from an evolutionary perspective. Sons need slightly
more energy to grow and tend to be bigger when they're born. They are less
likely to survive if they are malnourished as children, and smaller men tend to
be less attractive as potential mates. So in times of plenty, it makes sense to
produce sons: If they survive, they have the potential to sire more grandchildren. When food is scarce, hardier daughters may be a better option.

The mineral content of the women's diet may have had an effect. Several
studies have shown that women who eat diets rich in salt and potassium
(found in bananas and spinach, among other things) are more likely to have
boys, while those eating lots of calcium (found in milk and dairy products)
and magnesium (found in nuts, seeds, and dark chocolate) are more likely to
have girls, although the reason is unclear.

You could try combining these methods. In a recent study, twenty-one
women who wanted to have girls were given kits to help them predict when
they were ovulating and were told to stop having sex two days before they
were due to ovulate. They ate diets high in calcium and magnesium and low
in sodium and potassium for nine weeks before trying to conceive. Sixteen
of the women gave birth to a daughter, suggesting that the method worked,
although the low number of women in the study means that it could have
been down to chance. Other studies found no effect.

Even if these methods work at a population level, there's no guarantee
that they will work for you; they may simply tip the balance slightly in your
favor. On an individual level, you may just have to get on with it and be happy
with what you get.

. 150 .
Do twins run in families?

Some people melt at the prospect of two identical babies who will always share a special bond, while others quake in horror. If you've dismissed the prospect of twins because no one else in your family has them, think again.

There are two types of twins: identical (monozygotic), who account for around a third of all twins; and nonidentical (dizygotic), who account for the remaining two thirds. Although nonidentical twins seem to run in families to some extent, identical twins (caused by an embryo splitting soon after fertilization) seem to be a completely random event.

Despite the name, identical twins aren't identical at all. Although they start out with the same genes, mutations creep in during the many rounds of cell division that enable a baby to grow, which explains why sometimes one twin develops a genetic disease when the other doesn't. Precisely where in the uterus the embryos implant can influence how much blood and how many toxins twins are exposed to, which can lead to differences in growth.

Nonidentical twins seem to run on the mother's side of the family, so if your mom or your sister had twins, you are twice as likely to have them as the average woman, possibly because there is some hereditary factor that causes more than one egg to be released each month at ovulation. The risk of having nonidentical twins quadruples with age, as the pool of remaining eggs begins to dwindle and the body produces more of the hormone that stimulates the ovaries to release eggs.

Although the number of identical twins born is relatively consistent around the world, the rate of dizygotic twinning varies widely, presumably because of genetic factors. In Nigeria, around one in every eleven newborns is a twin, while in Japan it is more like one in every two hundred and fifty. In the U.S. and Europe, between ten and twenty in every thousand births results in a twin.

Identical twins seem to be more common in women undergoing IVF, even if they have only one embryo transferred. This may have something to do with the physical processes involved in IVF or the way embryos are cultured before implantation. One recent study hinted that identical twins were more likely to form if there were structural weaknesses in the very early embryo.

This happened to one of my colleagues, who already had one child through IVF and hoped to have a second by implanting one of the remaining embryos. She was shown a photo of her defrosted embryo shortly before it was implanted, then had a scan four weeks later, only to be confronted with two embryos sitting side by side in her uterus. Just imagine being able to sit with your twin and see a photo of yourself when you were one individual rather than two.

ACKNOWLEDGMENTS

The original seeds of this book were planted at *New Scientist,* so I must thank my colleagues, in particular Richard Fisher, Rowan Hooper, and Sumit Paul-Choudhury, for encouraging me to write and develop the "Bumpology" column in the first place.

Thanks also to the great friends I made through the National Childbirth Trust: Natalie Moore, Janet Hanson, Rhona Cairns, Liz Foley, Hanna Gronborg, and Michelle Ellis, for keeping me sane during the early baby days and providing an ongoing source of questions and inspiration for this book. I am also indebted to Laura Gallagher, Nicola Jones, and Clemmie Hooper, who gave up their time to read various drafts of the book and offered their feedback as mothers, editors, and midwives.

I would also like to pay homage to my Facebook Bumpologists: Betony Bennett, Eloise Hansell, Amy Frary, Jo Marchant, Tim Boucher, Vicky Sumner, Joanna Hurley, Angelica Ronald, and Joanna Hill—moms and dads who contributed their own questions about pregnancy and babies and provided a sounding board at various stages of the book's development.

I have picked many brains during the writing of *Bumpology,* and I am extremely grateful to the many researchers, doctors, and other health workers—both quoted and unquoted—who patiently talked me through their research and unflinchingly responded to some of the quirkier questions I posed. I must give particular thanks to Philip Steer and Maria Elliott for sparing me so much of their time and expertise.

I'd also like to thank Susanna Wadeson and her colleagues at Bantam Press for their encouragement during the writing of this book, and Mark Henderson for telling Susanna about "Bumpology" in the first place. Similarly, I must thank Patrick Barkham for introducing me to my excellent agent, Karolina Sutton at Curtis Brown, whose support has been invaluable.

Finally, thanks to my husband, Nic Fleming, for his patience and childcare wizardry, without whom this adventure in baby-making never would have been possible; and to our children, Matilda and Max, whose growth and development have provided me with so much inspiration and joy.

notes

Foreword

Sense About Science, Straight Statistics. *Making sense of statistics*. 2010. Available from: http://www.senseaboutscience.org/data/files/resources/1/MSofStatistics.pdf.

One: Bump
Food and drink

Why do pregnant women crave unhealthy food?

BabyCenter [Internet]. Food cravings and what they mean. Available from: http://www.babycenter.com/0_food-cravings-and-what-they-mean_1313971.bc.

Faas MM, Melgert BN, de Vos P. A brief review on how pregnancy and sex hormones interfere with taste and food intake. *Chemosen Percept*. 2010;3(1):51–6.

Davidsen L, Vistisen B, Astrup A. Impact of the menstrual cycle on determinants of energy balance: a putative role in weight-loss attempts. *Int J Obes (Lond)*. 2007;31:1777–85.

Gibson EL, Wainwright CJ, Booth DA. Disguised protein in lunch after low-protein breakfast conditions food-flavor preferences dependent on recent lack of protein intake. *Physiol Behav*. 1995;58(2):363–71.

BBC News. Pregnancy cravings "on the rise." 2008 Apr 26. Available from: http://news.bbc.co.uk/1/hi/health/7370524.stm.

Do pregnant women really eat coal?

Young SL. Pica in pregnancy: new ideas about an old condition. *Annu Rev Nutr.* 2010;30:403–22.

What causes morning sickness?

Verberg MF, Gillott DJ, Al-Fardan N, Grudzinskas JG. Hyperemesis gravidarium, a literature review. *Hum Reprod Update.* 2005;11(5):527–39.

Yaron Y, Lehavi O, Orr-Urtreger A, Gull I, Lessing JB, Amit A, Ben-Yosef D. Maternal serum HCG is higher in the presence of a female fetus as early as week three post-fertilization. *Hum Reprod.* 2002;17(2):485–9.

Flaxman SM, Sherman PW. Morning sickness: a mechanism for protecting mother and embryo. *Q Rev Biol.* 2000;77(2):113–48.

Bainbridge, D. *A visitor within: the science of pregnancy.* London: Weidenfeld and Nicolson; 2000.

Is there anything I can do to reduce morning sickness?

National Institute for Health and Clinical Excellence. Antenatal care: routine care for the healthy pregnant woman. 2008. Available from: http://www.nice.org.uk/CG62.

American College of Obstetricians and Gynecologists. Practice bulletin: nausea and vomiting of pregnancy. *Obstet Gynecol.* 2004;103(4):803–14.

Matthews A, Dowswell T, Haas DM, Doyle M, O'Mathúna DP. Interventions for nausea and vomiting in early pregnancy. *Cochrane Database Syst Rev.* 2010;9:CD007575.

How much alcohol is it safe to drink during pregnancy?

Henderson J, Gray R, Brocklehurst P. Systematic review of effects of low-moderate prenatal alcohol exposure on pregnancy outcome. *BJOG.* 2007 Jul;114(3):243–52.

Royal College of Obstetricians and Gynaecologists. Alcohol and pregnancy: information for you. 2006; Jan 11. Available from: http://www.rcog.org.uk/womens-health/clinical-guidance/alcohol-and-pregnancy-information-you.

Kelly Y, Sacker A, Gray R, Kelly J, Wolke D, Quigley MA. Light drinking in pregnancy, a risk for behavioural problems and cognitive deficits at 3 years of age? *In J Epidemiol.* 2009;38(1):129–40.

Kelly Y, Iacovou M, Quigley MA, Gray R, Wolke D, Kelly J, Sacker A. Light drinking versus abstinence in pregnancy—behavioural and cognitive outcomes in 7-year-old children: a longitudinal cohort study. *BJOG.* 2013 Oct;120(11):1340–7.

Kesmodel US, Bertrand J, Støvring H, Skarpness B, Denny CH, Mortensen EL; Lifestyle During Pregnancy Study Group. The effect of different alcohol drinking patterns in early to mid-pregnancy on the child's intelligence, attention, and executive function. *BJOG*. 2012 Sep;119(10):1180–90.

Gavaghan C. "You can't *handle* the truth"; medical paternalism and prenatal alcohol use. *J Med Ethics*. 2009;35:300–3.

Feldman HS, Jones KL, Lindsay S, Slymen D, Klonoff-Cohen H, Kao K, Rao S, Chambers C. Prenatal alcohol exposure patterns and alcohol-related birth defects and growth deficiencies: a prospective study. *Alcoholism Clin Exp Res*. 2012 Apr;36(4):670–6.

Can unborn babies taste what Mom is eating?

Mennella JA, Johnson A, Beauchamp GK. Garlic ingestion by pregnant women alters the odor of amniotic fluid. *Chem Senses*. 1995 Apr;20(2):207–9.

Beauchamp GK, Mennella JA. Flavor perception in human infants: development and functional significance. *Digestion*. 2011;83 Suppl. 1:1–6.

Mennella JA, Jagnow CP, Beauchamp GK. Prenatal and postnatal flavor learning by human infants. *Pediatrics*. 2001 Jun 1;107:e88.

Can Mom's food fads influence her baby's palate?

Abate P, Pueta M, Spear NE, Molina JC. Fetal learning about ethanol and later ethanol responsiveness: evidence against "safe" amounts of prenatal exposure. *Exp Biol Med*. 2008 Feb;233(2):139–54.

Eade AM, Youngentob SL. The interaction of gestational and postnatal ethanol experience on the adolescent and adult odor-mediated responses to ethanol in observer and demonstrator rats. *Alcohol Clin Exp Res*. 2010 Oct;34(10):1705–13.

Crystal SR, Bernstein IL. Infant salt preference and mothers' morning sickness. *Appetite*. 1998 Jun;30(3):297–307.

Is coffee bad for my baby?

Jahanfar S, Sharifah H. Effects of restricted caffeine intake by mother on fetal, neonatal and pregnancy outcome. *Cochrane Database Syst Rev*. 2009 April 15:2:CD006965.

Bakker R, Steegers EA, Obradov A, Raat H, Hofman A, Jaddoe VW. Maternal caffeine intake from coffee and tea, fetal growth, and the risks of adverse birth outcomes: the Generation R Study. *Am J Clin Nutr*. 2010 Jun;91(6):1691–8.

Crozier TW, Stalmach A, Lean ME, Crozier A. Espresso coffees, caffeine and chlorogenic acid intake: potential health implications. *Food Funct.* 2012;3:30–3.

UK Food Standards Agency. *Eating while you are pregnant.* 2002.

Can I eat peanuts during pregnancy?

Sicherer SH, Wood RA, Stablein D, Lindblad R, Burks AW, Liu AH, Jones SM, Fleischer DM, Leung DY, Sampson HA. Maternal consumption of peanut during pregnancy is associated with peanut sensitization in atopic infants. *J Allergy Clin Immunol.* 2010 Dec 1;126(6):1191–7.

Committee on Toxicology of Chemicals in Food, Consumer Products and the Environment. Statement on the review of the 1998 COT recommendations of peanut avoidance. COT Statement 2008/7. 2008;Dec. Available from http://cot.food.gov.uk/pdfs/cotstatement200807peanut.pdf.

Greer FR, Sicherer SH, Burks AW; American Academy of Pediatrics Committee on Nutrition; American Academy of Pediatrics Section on Allergy and Immunology. Effects of early nutritional interventions on the development of atopic disease in infants and children: the role of maternal dietary restriction, breast-feeding, timing of introduction of complementary foods, and hydrolyzed formulas. *Pediatrics.* 2008 Jan 1;121(1):183–91.

Should pregnant women really eat for two?

McDonald SD, Pullenayegum E, Taylor VH, Lutsiv O, Bracken K, Good C, Hutton E, Sword W. Despite 2009 guidelines, few women report being counselled correctly about weight gain during pregnancy. *Am J Obstet Gynecol.* 2011;205(333):e1–6.

Nehring I, Schmoll S, Beyerlein A, Hauner H, von Kries R. Gestational weight gain and long-term postpartum weight retention: a meta-analysis. *Am J Clin Nutr.* 2011 Nov;94(5):1225–31.

American Pregnancy Association. Eating for two when over- or underweight. 2011 Jun. Available from: http://www.americanpregnancy.org/pregnancyhealth/eatingfortwo.html.

How dangerous is it to eat Camembert and blue cheese?

National Health Service. Listeriosis. 2013 Jan 17. Available from: http://www.nhs.uk/conditions/listeriosis/Pages/Introduction.aspx.

Lamont RF, Sobel J, Mazaki-Tovi S, Kusanovic JP, Vaisbuch E, Kim SK, Uldbjerg N, Romero R. Listeriosis in human pregnancy: a systematic review. *J Perinat Med.* 2011 May;39(3):227–36.

Jackson KA, Iwamoto M, Swerdlow D. Pregnancy-associated listeriosis. *Epidemiol Infect*. 2010 Oct;38(10):1503–9.

Varma JK, Samuel MC, Marcus R, Hoekstra RM, Medus C, Segler S, Anderson BJ, Jones TF, Shiferaw B, Haubert N, Megginson M, McCarthy PV, Graves L, Gilder TV, Angulo FJ. *Listeria monocytogenes* infection from foods prepared in a commercial establishment: a case-control study of potential sources of sporadic illness in the United States. *Clin Infect Dis*. 2007;44(4):521–8.

Little CL, Pires SM, Gillespie IA, Grant K, Nichols GL. Attribution of human listeria monocytogenes infections in England and Wales to ready-to-eat food sources placed on the market: adaptation of the Hald salmonella source attribution model. *Foodborne Pathog Dis*. 2010;7(7):749–56.

The Pregnant Body

Can the shape of my bump or anything else predict the gender of my child?

Perry DF, DiPietro J, Costigan K. Are women carrying "basketballs" really having boys? Testing pregnancy folklore. *Birth*. 1999 Sep;26(3):172–7.

Askling J, Erlandsson G, Kaijser M, Akre O, Ekbom A. Sickness in pregnancy and sex of child. *Lancet*. 1999;354(9195):2053.

James WH. Hyperemesis gravidarum and sex of child. *Lancet*. 2000 Jan 29;355(9201):407.

McKenna DS, Ventolini G, Neiger R, Downing C. "Gender-related differences in fetal heart rate during first trimester. *Fetal Diagn Ther*. 2006;21:144–7.

Dawes NW, Dawes GS, Moulden M, Redman CW. Fetal heart rate patterns in term labor vary with sex, gestational age, epidural analgesia, and fetal weight. *Am J Obstet Gynecol*. 1999 Jan;180(1):181–7.

Tamimi RM, Lagiou P, Mucci LA, Hsieh CC, Adami HO, Trichopoulos D. Average energy intake among pregnant women carrying a boy compared with a girl. *BMJ*. 2003 June 7;326(7401):1245–6.

Ramzi S. The relationship between placental location and fetal gender (Ramzi's method). 2011 Jun 14. Available from: http://hcp.obgyn.net/urogynecology/content/article/1760982/1878451.

Demissie K, Breckenridge MB, Joseph L, Rhoads GG. Placenta previa: preponderance of male sex at birth. *Am J Epidemiol*. 1999 May 1;149(9):824–30.

The S, Chan L. The role of placental location assessment in the prediction of fetal gender. *Ultrasound Obstet Gynecol*. 2010;36:242.

Why don't pregnant women topple over?

Whitcome KK, Shapiro LJ, Lieberman DE. Fetal load and the evolution of lumbar lordosis in bipedal hominins. *Nature*. 2007 Dec 13;450(7172):1075.

Why do women get a linea nigra and other brown patches on their skin during pregnancy?

Muallem MM, Rubeiz NG. Physiological and biological skin changes in pregnancy. *Clin Dermatol*. 2006 Mar-Apr;24(2):80–3.

Elling SV, Powell FC. Physiological changes in the skin during pregnancy. *Clin Dermatol*. 1997 Jan-Feb;15(1):35–43.

Is there anything I can do to prevent stretch marks?

Lurie S, Matas Z, Fux A, Golan A, Sadan O. Association of serum relaxin with striae gravidarum in pregnant women. *Arch Gynecol Obstet*. 2011 Feb;283(2):219–22.

Taavoni S, Soltanipour F, Haghani H, Ansarian H, Kheirkhah M. Effects of olive oil on striae gravidarum in the second trimester of pregnancy. *Complement Ther Clin Pract*. 2011 Aug;17(3):167–9.

Buchanan K, Fletcher HM, Reid M. Prevention of striae gravidarum with cocoa butter cream. *Int J Gynaecol Obstet*. 2010 Jan;108(1):65–8.

Osman H, Usta IM, Rubeiz N, Abu-Rustum R, Charara I, Nassar AH. Cocoa-butter lotion for prevention of striae gravidarum: a double-blind, randomized and placebo-controlled trial. *BJOG*. 2008 Aug;115(9):1138–42.

Young G, Jewell D. Creams for preventing stretch marks in pregnancy. *Cochrane Database Syst Rev*. 1996;1:CD000066.

Do big parents have bigger babies?

Peregrine E, Peebles D. Fetal growth and growth restriction. *Fetal Medicine: Basic Science and Clinical Practice* London: Churchill; 2008.

Johansson K, Linne Y, Rossner S, Neovius M. Maternal predictors of birthweight: the importance of weight gain during pregnancy. *Obesity Res Clin Pract*. 2007 Dec;1(4):243–52.

Does a woman's body shape permanently change after pregnancy?

Lassek WD, Gaulin SJ. Changes in body-fat distribution in relation to parity in American women: a covert form of maternal depletion. *Am J Phys Anthropo*. 2006;131:295–302.

Can Jacuzzis and saunas really cause miscarriage?

Chambers CD. Risks of hyperthermia associated with hot tub or spa use by pregnant women. *Birth Defects Res A Clin Mol Teratol*. 2006 Aug;76(8):569–73.

American Pregnancy Association. Pregnant in a hot tub. 2013 Jan. Available from: http://www.americanpregnancy.org/pregnancyhealth/hottubs.htm.

Why do so many human embryos miscarry before twelve weeks?

Vanneste E, Voet T, Le Caignec C, Ampe M, Konings P, Melotte C, Debrock S, Amyere M, Vikkula M, Schuit F, Fryns JP, Verbeke G, D'Hooghe T, Moreau Y, Vermeesch JR. Chromosome instability is common in human cleavage-stage embryos. *Nat Med*. 2009;15:577–83.

Wilcox AJ, Weinberg CR, O'Connor JF, Baird DD, Schlatterer JP, Canfield RE, Armstrong EG, Nisula BC. Incidence of early loss of pregnancy. *New Engl J Med*. 1988 July 28;319(4):189–94.

Royal College of Obstetricians and Gynaecologists. Early miscarriage: information for you. 2008 Jan 1. Available from: http://www.rcog.org.uk/womens-health/clinical-guidance/early-miscarriage-information-you.

Regan L, Braude PR, Trembath PL. Influence of past reproductive performance on risk of spontaneous abortion. *BMJ*. 1989;229:545–9.

IVF Authority [blog]. IVF: Commonly asked questions, fears and concerns—part 4: what are my chances and how many times should I try? Available from: http://www.ivfauthority.com/2011/02/ivf-commonly-asked-questions-fears-and_09.html.

Exercise

Is it safe to exercise during pregnancy?

Kramer MS, McDonald SW. Aerobic exercise for women during pregnancy. *Cochrane Database Syst Rev*. 2006;3:CD000180.

Madsen M, Jørgensen T, Jensen ML, Juhl M, Olsen J, Andersen PK, Nybo Andersen AM. Leisure time physical exercise during pregnancy and the risk of miscarriage: a study within the Danish National Birth Cohort. *BJOG*. 2007 Nov 1;114(11):1419–26.

Haakstad LA, Bø K. Exercise in pregnant women and birth weight: a randomized controlled trial. *BMC Pregnancy Childbirth*. 2011 Sep 30;11:66.

Clapp JF 3rd. Exercise during pregnancy. A clinical update. *Clin Sports Med.* 2000 Apr;19(2):273–86.

May LE, Glaros A, Yeh HW, Clapp JF 3rd, Gustafson KM. Aerobic exercise during pregnancy influences fetal cardiac autonomic control of heart rate and heart rate variability. *Early Hum Dev.* 2010 April;86(4):213–17.

Szymanski LM, Satin AJ. Strenuous exercise in pregnancy: is there a limit? *Am J Obstet Gynecol.* 2012 Jan;206(1):S71.

Szymanski LM, Satin AJ. A prospective investigation of the U.S. public health recommendations for physical activity during pregnancy. *Am J Obstet Gynecol.* 2012 Jan;206(1):S71–S72.

What stomach exercises can I do when pregnant?

Henderson C, Macdonald S, eds. *Mayes' midwifery: a textbook for midwives.* 13th ed. London: Baillière Tindall; 2004.

Will lying on my back harm my baby?

Rossi A, Cornette J, Johnson MR, Karamermer Y, Springeling T, Opic P, Moelker A, Krestin GP, Steegers E, Roos-Hesselink J, van Geuns RJ. Quantitative cardiovascular magnetic resonance in pregnant women: cross-sectional analysis of physiological parameters throughout pregnancy and the impact of the supine position. *J Cardiovas Magn Reson.* 2011 June 27;13:31.

Do pelvic-floor exercises actually work?

Hay-Smith J, Mørkved S, Fairbrother KA, Herbison GP. Pelvic floor muscle training for prevention and treatment of urinary and faecal incontinence in antenatal and postnatal women *Cochrane Database Syst Rev.* 2008;4:CD007471.

Citak N, Cam C, Arslan H, Karateke A, Tug N, Ayaz R, Celik C. Postpartum sexual function of women and the effects of early pelvic-floor-muscle exercises. *Acta Obstet Gynecol Scand.* 2010;89:817–22.

Guy's and St. Thomas' NHS Foundation Trust. Pelvic floor exercises for women. 2010. Available from: http://www.guysandstthomas.nhs.uk/resources/patient -information/maternity/pelvic-floor-exercises-for-women.pdf.

Baby on the Brain

Does pregnancy make women forgetful?

Glynn NM. Giving birth to a new brain: hormone exposures of pregnancy influence human memory. *Psychoneuroendocrinology.* 2010 Sept.;35(8):1148–55.

Oatridge A, Holdcroft A, Saeed N, Hajnal JV, Puri BK, Fusi L, Bydder GM. Change in brain size during and after pregnancy: study in healthy women and women with preeclampsia. *Am J Neuroradiol*. 2002;23:19–26.

Kinsley CH, Trainer R, Stafisso-Sandoz G, Quadros P, Marcus LK, Hearon C, Meyer EA, Hester N, Morgan M, Kozub FJ, Lambert KG. Motherhood and the hormones of pregnancy modify concentrations of hippocampal neuronal dendritic spines. *Horm Behav*. 2006 Mar;49(2):131–42.

Kinsley CH, Madonia L, Gifford GW, Tureski K, Griffin GR, Lowry C, Williams J, Collins J, McLearie H, Lambert KG. Motherhood improves learning and memory. *Nature*. 1999 Nov 11;401:137–8.

Pearson RM, Lightman SL, Evans J. Emotional sensitivity for motherhood: late pregnancy is associated with enhanced accuracy to encode emotional faces. *Horm Behav*. 2009 Nov;56(5):557–63.

Entringer S, Buss C, Shirtcliff EA, Cammack AL, Yim IS, Chicz-DeMet A, Sandman CA, Wadhwa PD. Attenuation of maternal psychophysiological stress responses and the maternal cortisol awakening response over the course of human pregnancy. *Stress*. 2010 May;13(3):258–68.

Is stress during pregnancy bad for my baby?

Hobel CJ, Goldstein A, Barrett ES. Psychosocial stress and pregnancy outcome. *Clin Obstet Gynecol*. 2008 Jun;51(2):333–48.

Littleton HL, Bye K, Buck K, Amacker A. Psychosocial stress during pregnancy and perinatal outcomes: a meta-analytic review. *J Psychosom Obstet Gynaecol*. 2010 Dec;31(4):219–28.

DiPietro JA, Kivlighan KT, Costigan KA, Rubin SE, Shiffler DE, Henderson JL, Pillion JP. Prenatal antecedents of newborn neurological maturation. *Child Devel*. 2010 Feb;81(1):115–30.

Storey AE, Walsh CJ, Quinton RL, Wynne-Edwards KE. Hormonal correlates of paternal responsiveness in new and expectant fathers. *Evol Hum Behav*. 2000 Mar 1;21(2):79–95.

Can men get pregnancy symptoms, too?

Brennan A, Ayers S, Ahmed H, Marshall-Lucette S. A critical review of the Couvade syndrome: the pregnant male. *J Reprod Infant Psychol*. 2007 Aug;25(3):173–89.

Kim P, Swain JE. Sad dads: paternal postpartum depression. *Psychiatry (Edgmont)*. 2007 Feb;4(2):35–47.

Why do women go into nesting overdrive in the final weeks of pregnancy?

Kim P, Leckman JF, Mayes LC, Feldman R, Wang X, Swain JE. The plasticity of human maternal brain: longitudinal changes in brain anatomy during the early postpartum period. *Behav Neurosci.* 2010 Oct;124(5):695–700.

Kim P, Feldman R, Mayes LC, Eicher V, Thompson N, Leckman JF, Swain JE. Breast-feeding, brain activation to own infant cry, and maternal sensitivity. *J Child Psychol Psychiatry.* 2011 Aug;52(8):907–15.

Are some women naturally more maternal than others?

Atzil S, Hendler T, Feldman R. Specifying the neurobiological basis of human attachment: brain, hormones, and behavior in synchronous and intrusive mothers. *Neuropsychopharmacology.* 2011 Dec;36(13):2603–15.

Do men change when they become dads?

Gordon I, Zagoory-Sharon O, Leckman JF, Feldman R. Prolactin, oxytocin, and the development of paternal behavior across the first six months of fatherhood. *Horm Behav.* 2010 Aug;58(3):513–8.

Feldman R, Gordon I, Schneiderman I, Weisman O, Zagoory-Sharon O. Natural variations in maternal and paternal care are associated with systematic changes in oxytocin following parent-infant contact. *Psychoneuroendocrinology.* 2010 Sep;35(8):1133–41.

Alvergne A, Faurie C, Raymond M. Variation in testosterone levels and male reproductive effort: Insight from a polygynous human population. *Horm Behav.* 2009 Nov;56(5):491–7.

Berg SJ, Wynne-Edwards KE. Changes in testosterone, cortisol, and estradiol levels in men becoming fathers. *Mayo Clin Proc.* 2001 Jun;76(6):582–92.

The Developing Baby

When does a baby become conscious?

Lagercrantz H. The emergence of the mind—a borderline of human viability? *Acta Paediatr.* 2007;96:327–8.

Lagercrantz H, Changeux JP. The emergence of human consciousness: from fetal to neonatal life. *Pediatr Res.* 2009;65(3):255–60.

Mellor DJ, Diesch TJ, Gunn AJ, Bennet L. Fetal "awareness" and "pain": what precautions should be taken to safeguard fetal welfare during experiments? *AATEX.* 2007;14(special issue):79–83.

Does a wriggly bump equal a boisterous baby?

Hayat TT, Nihat A, Martinez-Biarge M, McGuinness A, Allsop JM, Hajnal JV, Rutherford MA. Optimization and initial experience of a multislice balanced steady-state free precession cine sequence for the assessment of fetal behavior in utero. *Am J Neuroradiol*. 2011;32:331–8.

Dipietro JA. Psychological and psychophysiological considerations regarding the maternal-fetal relationship. *Infant Child Devel*. 2010 Jan;19(1):27–38.

DiPietro JA, Bornstein MH, Costigan KA, Pressman EK, Hahn CS, Painter K, Smith BA, Yi LJ. What does fetal movement predict about behavior during the first two years of life? *Devel Psychobiol*. 2002 May;40(4):358–71.

St. James-Roberts I, Menon-Johansson P. Predicting infant crying from fetal movement data: an exploratory study. *Early Hum Dev*. 1999;54:55–62.

Degani S, Leibovitz Z, Shapiro I, Ohel G. Twins' temperament: early prenatal sonographic assessment and postnatal correlation. *J Perinatol*. 2009 May;29(5):337–42.

Can a baby detect its mother's mood?

Araki M, Nishitani S, Ushimaru K, Masuzaki H, Oishi K, Shinohara K. Fetal response to induced maternal emotions. *J Physiol Sci*. 2010;60(3):213–20.

DiPietro JA, Ghera MM, Costigan KA. Prenatal origins of temperamental reactivity. *Early Hum Dev*. 2008 Sep;84(9):569–75.

What do babies learn during their time in the womb?

Hepper P. Fetal psychology: an embryonic science. In: Nijhuis J, ed. *Fetal Behavior—Developmental and Perinatal Aspects*. London: Oxford University Press; 1992.

Hepper PG. Fetal memory: Does it exist? What does it do? *Acta Paediatr Suppl*. 1996;416:16–20.

Dirix CE, Nijhuis JG, Jongsma HW, Hornstra G. Aspects of fetal learning and memory. *Child Dev*. 2009;80(4):1251–8.

Will playing Mozart to my bump make my baby more intelligent?

Shetler DJ. Prelude to a musical life: prenatal music experiences. *Music Educators J*. 1985;71(7):26–7.

McLachlan JC. Music and spatial task performance. *Nature*. 1993 Oct 14;365(6447):611.

Rauscher FH, Robinson KD, Jens JJ. Improved maze learning through early music exposure in rats. *Neurol Res*. 1998 Jul;20(5):427–32.

Al-Qahtani NH. Foetal response to music and voice. *Aust N Z J Obstet Gynaecol.* 2005 Oct;45(5):414–17.

Lubetzky R, Mimouni FB, Dollberg S, Reifen R, Ashbel G, Mandel D. Effect of music by Mozart on energy expenditure in growing preterm infants. *Pediatrics.* 2010 Jan;125(1):24–8.

Will my baby look like Mom or Dad?

White D, Rabago-Smith M. Genotype-phenotype associations and human eye color. *J Hum Genet.* 2011;56:5–7.

Johannsdottir B, Thorarinsson F, Thordarson A, Magnusson TE. Heritability of craniofacial characteristics between parents and offspring estimated from lateral cephalograms. *Am J Orthod Dentofacial Orthop,* 2005 Feb;127(2):200–7.

Chang C, Miyazono H, Komiya T, Nakasima A. The similarity between parents and offspring in facial soft tissue: a frontal-view study. *Aust Orthod J.* 1998 Mar;15(2):85–92.

Gelgör IE, Karaman AI, Zekiç E. The use of parental data to evaluate soft tissues in an Anatolian Turkish population according to Holdaway soft tissue norms. *Am J Orthod Dentofacial Orthop.* 2006 Mar;129(3):330.e1–330.e9.

Alford JR. Are political orientations genetically transmitted? *Am Pol Sci Rev.* 2005;99(2):153–67.

Do unborn babies dream?

Walusinski O. Fetal yawning. *Front Neurol Neurosci.* 2010;28:32–41.

Hobson JA. REM sleep and dreaming: towards a theory of protoconsciousness. *Nat Rev Neurosci.* 2009 Nov;10:803–14.

Mirmiran M, Maas YG, Ariagno RL. Development of fetal neonatal sleep and circadian rhythms. *Sleep Med Rev.* 2003;7(4):321–34.

Serón-Ferré M, Mendez N, Abarzua-Catalan L, Vilches N, Valenzuela FJ, Reynolds HE, Llanos AJ, Rojas A, Valenzuela GJ, Torres-Farfan C. Circadian rhythms in the fetus. *Mol Cell Endocrinol.* 2012;349:68–75.

Are babies more active at night?

Mirmiran M, Maas YG, Ariagno RL. Development of fetal neonatal sleep and circadian rhythms. *Sleep Med Rev.* 2003;7(4):321–34.

How do fingerprints develop?

Langenburg G. Are one's fingerprints similar to those of his or her parents in any discernable way? *Scientific American.* 2005 Jan 24. Available from:

http://www.scientificamerican.com/article.cfm?id=are-ones-fingerprints-sim.

Kücken M, Newell AC. Fingerprint formation. *J Theor Biol*. 2005 Jul 7;235(1):71–83.

Kahn HS, Graff M, Stein AD, Zybert PA, McKeague IW, Lumey LH. A fingerprint characteristic associated with the early prenatal environment. *Am J Hum Biol*. 2008;20:59–65.

Kahn HS, Graff M, Stein AD, Lumey LH. A fingerprint marker from early gestation associated with diabetes in middle age: the Dutch Hunger Winter families study. *Int J Epidemiol*. 2009;38:101–9.

Two: Birth
Get a Move On

Who decides when it's time to come out?

Bainbridge D. *A Visitor Within: The Science of Pregnancy*. London: Weidenfeld and Nicolson; 2000.

Golightly E, Jabbour HN, Norman JE. Endocrine immune interactions in human parturition. *Mol Cell Endocrinol*. 2011 Mar 15;335(1):52–9.

Mitchell BF, Taggart MJ. Are animal models relevant to key aspects of human parturition? *Am J Physiol Regul Integr Comp Physiol*. 2009 Sep;297(3):R525–45.

Can my state of mind delay labor?

Lew BR, Chung PH, Slade MD. Influence of Valentine's Day and Halloween on birth timing. *Soc Sci Med*. 2011 Oct;73(8):1246–8.

Is it normal for pregnancies to run past their due date?

Baskett TF, Nagele F. Naegele's rule: a reappraisal. *BJOG*. 2000 Nov;107(11):1433–5.

The length of uncomplicated human gestation. *Obstet Gynecol*. 1990 Jun;75(6):929–32.

Balchin I, Whittaker JC, Lamont RF, Steer PJ. Timing of planned Cesarean delivery by racial group. *Obstet Gynecol*. 2008;111(3):659–66.

NCT evidence-based briefing: induction of labor. *New Digest*. 2002 Feb.

Can curry or anything else help trigger labor?

Hall HG, McKenna LG, Griffiths DL. Complementary and alternative medicine for induction of labor. *Women and Birth*. 2012 Sep;25(3):142–8.

Holst L, Haavik S, Nordeng H. Raspberry leaf—should it be recommended to pregnant women? *Complement Ther Clin Pract*. 2009;15:204–8.

Does having a membrane sweep work?

Boulvain M, Stan CM, Irion O. Membrane sweeping for induction of labor. *Cochrane Database Syst Rev.* 2005;1:CD000451.

Will being induced mean I'm less likely to have a natural birth?

Hilder L, Costeloe K, Thilaganathan B. Prolonged pregnancy: evaluating gestation-specific risks of fetal and infant mortality. *BJOG.* 1998 Feb;105(2):169–73.

Caughey AB, Sundaram V, Kaimal AJ, Gienger A, Cheng YW, McDonald KM, Shaffer BL, Owens DK, Bravata DM. Systematic review: elective induction of labor versus expectant management of pregnancy. *Ann Intern Med.* 2009 Aug 18;151(4):252–63.

Sanchez-Ramos L, Olivier F, Delke I, Kaunitz AM. Labor induction versus expectant management for postterm pregnancies: a systematic review with meta-analysis. *Obstet Gynecol.* 2003 Jun;101(6):1312–18.

Gülmezoglu AM, Crowther CA, Middleton P. Induction of labor for improving birth outcomes for women at or beyond term. *Cochrane Database Syst Rev.* 2006;4:CD004945.

Hermus MA, Verhoeven CJ, Mol BW, de Wolf GS, Fiedeldeij CA. Comparison of induction of labor and expectant management in postterm pregnancy: a matched cohort study. *J Midwifery Womens Health.* 2009;54(5):351–6.

Wei SQ, Luo ZC, Xu H, Fraser WD. The effect of early oxytocin augmentation in labor: a meta-analysis. *Obstet Gynecol.* 2009 Sep;114(3):641–9.

Wei SQ, Luo ZC, Qi HP, Xu H, Fraser WD. High-dose vs low-dose oxytocin for labor augmentation: a systematic review. *Am J Obstet Gynecol.* 2010 Oct;203(4):296–304.

Will rocking on my hands and knees cause my baby to turn over?

Matsuo K, Shimoya K, Ushioda N, Kimura T. Maternal positioning and fetal positioning in utero. *J Obstet Gynaecol Res.* 2007 Jun;33(3):279–82.

Zhao XB, Shan JZ. [Changing fetal position through maternal posture.] *Zhonghua Fu Chan Ke Za Zhi.* 1993 Sep;28(9):517–19.

Hunter S, Hofmeyr GJ, Kulier R. Hands and knees posture in late pregnancy or labor for fetal malposition (lateral or posterior). *Cochrane Database Syst Rev.* 2007;4:CD001063.

National Institute for Health and Clinical Excellence. Caesarean section. NICE clinical guideline (CG132). 2011 Nov.

Can I take a bath once my water has broken?

Eriksson M, Ladfors L, Mattsson LA, Fall O. Warm tub bath during labor. A study of 1,385 women with prelabor rupture of the membranes after 34 weeks of gestation. *Acta Obstet Gynecol Scand.* 1996 Aug;75(7):642–4.

The Big Push

Why do humans find it so difficult to give birth?

Rosenberg K. Bipedalism and human birth: the obstetrical dilemma revisited. *Evolutionary Anthropol.* 2005;4(5):161–8.

Is there any way to predict how long labor will last?

Neal JL, Lowe NK, Ahijevych KL, Patrick TE, Cabbage LA, Corwin EJ. "Active labor": duration and dilation rates among low-risk, nulliparous women with spontaneous labor onset: a systematic review. *J Midwifery Womens Health.* 2010;55(4):308–18.

Handa VL, Lockhart ME, Fielding JR, Bradley CS, Brubaker L, Cundiff GW, Ye W, Richter HE; Pelvic Floor Disorders Network. Racial differences in pelvic anatomy by magnetic resonance imaging. *Obstet Gynecol.* 2008;111(4):914–20.

Gurewitsch ED, Johnson E, Allen RH, Diament P, Fong J, Weinstein D, Chervenak FA. The descent curve of the grand multiparous woman. *Am J Obstet Gynecol.* 2003;189(4):1036–41.

Norman S, Tuuli M, Odibo A, Caughey A, Roehl K, Cahill A. Obese women have longer duration of first stage of labor. *Am J Obstet Gynecol.* 2012;206(1):S149–50.

Mahmood TA, Campbell DM, Wilson AW. Maternal height, shoe size, and outcome of labor in white primigravidas: a prospective anthropometric study. *BMJ.* 1988 Aug 20–27;297:515–17.

Dencker A, Berg M, Bergqvist L, Lilja H. Identification of latent phase factors associated with active labor duration in low-risk nulliparous women with spontaneous contractions. *Acta Obstet Gynecol Scand.* 2010;89:1034–9.

Are vaginal births really better than C-sections?

Listening to Mothers II: Report of the Second National U.S. Survey of Women's Childbearing Experiences. New York: Childbirth Connection; 2006.

McCourt C, Weaver J, Statham H, Beake S, Gamble J, Creedy DK. Elective cesarean section and decision-making: a critical review of the literature. *Birth*. 2007 Mar;34(1):65–79.

Benedetto C, Marozio L, Prandi G, Roccia A, Blefari S, Fabris C. Short-term maternal and neonatal outcomes by mode of delivery: a case-controlled study. *Eur J Obstet Gynecol Reprod Biol*. 2007 Nov;135(1):35–40.

A vaginal birth is harder on your sex life

Hicks TL, Goodall SF, Quattrone EM, Lydon-Rochelle MT. Postpartum sexual functioning and method of delivery: summary of the evidence. *J Midwifery Womens Health*. 2004;49(5):430–6.

Rathfisch G, Dikencik BK, Kizilkaya Beji N, Comert N, Tekirdag AI, Kadioglu A. Effects of perineal trauma on postpartum sexual function. *J Adv Nurs*. 2010;66(12):2640–9.

Barrett G, Pendry E, Peacock J, Victor C, Thakar R, Manyonda I. Women's sexual health after childbirth. *BJOG*. 2000;107(2):186–95.

van Brummen HJ, Bruinse HW, van de Pol G, Heintz AP, van der Vaart CH. Which factors determine the sexual function 1 year after childbirth? *BJOG*. 2006 Aug;113(8):914–18.

Signorello LB, Harlow BL, Chekos AK, Repke JT. Postpartum sexual functioning and its relationship to perineal trauma: a retrospective cohort study of primiparous women. *Am J Obstet Gynecol*. 2001;184(5):881–90.

Vaginal births increase the risk of incontinence

National Institute for Health and Clinical Excellence. Caesarean section. NICE clinical guideline (CG132). 2011 Nov.

Press JZ, Klein MC, Kaczorowski J, Liston RM, von Dadelszen P. Does cesarean section reduce postpartum urinary incontinence? A systematic review. *Birth*. 2007 Sep;34(3):228–37.

It takes longer to recover after a C-section

Lydon-Rochelle MT, Holt VL, Martin DP. Delivery method and self-reported postpartum general health status among primiparous women. *Paediatr Perinat Epidemiol*. 2001;15(3):232–40.

National Institute for Health and Clinical Excellence. Caesarean section. NICE clinical guideline (CG132). 2011 Nov.

C-sections make it harder to bond with your baby

Cook E. Women who have caesareans "less likely to bond." *Daily Mail*. 2006 Jul 13.

Tulman LJ. Initial handling of newborn infants by vaginally and cesarean-delivered mothers. *Nurs Res.* 1986 Sep-Oct;35(5):296–300.

Swain JE, Tasgin E, Mayes LC, Feldman R, Constable RT, Leckman JF. Maternal brain response to own baby-cry is affected by caesarean-section delivery. *J Child Psychol Psychiatry.* 2008;49(10):1042–52.

Kim P, Feldman R, Mayes LC, Eicher V, Thompson N, Leckman JF, Swain JE. Breast-feeding, brain activation to own infant cry, and maternal sensitivity. *J Child Psychol Psychiatry.* 2011 Aug;52(8):907–15.

Durik AM, Hyde JS, Clark R. Sequelae of cesarean and vaginal deliveries: psychosocial outcomes for mothers and infants. *Dev Psychol.* 2000 Mar;36(2):251–60.

Winberg J. Mother and newborn baby: mutual regulation of physiology and behavior—a selective review. *Dev Psychobiol.* 2005 Nov;47(3):217–29.

C-sections make breast-feeding more difficult

Zanardo V, Svegliado G, Cavallin F, Giustardi A, Cosmi E, Litta P, Trevisanuto D. Elective cesarean delivery: does it have a negative effect on breast-feeding? *Birth.* 2010 Dec;37(4):275–9.

Hung KJ, Berg O. Early skin-to-skin after cesarean to improve breast-feeding. *MCN Am J Matern Child Nurs.* 2011 Sep-Oct;36(5):318–24; quiz 325–6.

Babies born by C-section are less healthy

National Institute for Health and Clinical Excellence. Caesarean section. NICE clinical guideline (CG132). 2011 Nov.

Thavagnanam S, Fleming J, Bromley A, Shields MD, Cardwell CR. A meta-analysis of the association between caesarean section and childhood asthma. *Clin Exp Allergy.* 2008 Apr;38(4):629–33.

Adams M, Doull I. Birth by caesarean section and asthma. *Clin Exper Allergy.* 2008 Apr;38(4):554–6.

Bager P, Wohlfahrt J, Westergaard T. Caesarean delivery and risk of atopy and allergic disease: meta-analyses. *Clin Exper Allergy.* 2008 Apr;38(4):634–42.

Are home births riskier than hospital births?

Royal College of Obstetricians and Gynaecologists/Royal College of Midwives. Home births. Joint statement no. 2. 2007 Apr.

National Collaborating Centre for Women's and Children's Health (UK). *Intrapartum care. Care of healthy women and their babies during childbirth.* London: RCOG Press; 2007.

Birthplace in England Collaborative Group, Brocklehurst P, Hardy P, Hollowell J, Linsell L, Macfarlane A, McCourt C, Marlow N, Miller A, Newburn M,

Petrou S, Puddicombe D, Redshaw M, Rowe R, Sandall J, Silverton L, Stewart M. Perinatal and maternal outcomes by planned place of birth for healthy women with low risk pregnancies: the Birthplace in England national prospective cohort study. *BMJ*. 2011 Nov 23;343:d7400.

NHS Choices. Home birth risk remains unclear. 2008 Apr 2. Available from: http://www.nhs.uk/news/2008/04April/Pages/Homebirthriskremainsunclear.aspx.

Does walking or squatting speed up labor?

Lawrence A, Lewis L, Hofmeyr GJ, Dowswell T, Styles C. Maternal positions and mobility during first-stage labor. *Cochrane Database Syst Rev*. 2009;2:CD003934.

Should I push?

Brancato RM, Church S, Stone PW. A meta-analysis of passive descent versus immediate pushing in nulliparous women with epidural analgesia in the second stage of labor. *J Obstet Gynecol Neonatal Nurs*. 2008 Jan-Feb;37(1):4–12.

Kelly M, Johnson E, Lee V, Massey L, Purser D, Ring K, Sanderson S, Styles J, Wood D. Delayed versus immediate pushing in second stage of labor. *MCN: Am J Matern Child Nurs*. 2010 Mar-Apr;35(2):81–8.

Is it better to tear or be cut in terms of healing?

Kalis V, Kettle C, Raisanen SH, de Leeuw JW, Jundt K, de Tayrac R, Jansova M, Ismail KM; perineal trauma PEERS group. Episiotomy characteristics and risks for obstetric anal sphincter injuries: a case-control study. *BJOG*. 2012 May;119(6):724–30.

Does perineal massage work?

Beckmann MM, Garrett AJ. Antenatal perineal massage for reducing perineal trauma. *Cochrane Database Syst Rev*. 2006;1:CD005123.

Oxford Radcliffe Hospitals NHS Trust. Antenatal perineal massage: information for women. 2011 Aug.

Is there anything else I can do to prevent tearing?

Aasheim V, Nilsen ABV, Lukasse M, Reinar LM. Perineal techniques during the second stage of labor for reducing perineal trauma. *Cochrane Database Syst Rev*. 2011;12:CD006672.

Will delaying cord-clamping benefit my baby?

Andersson O, Hellström-Westas L, Andersson D, Domellöf M. Effect of delayed versus early umbilical cord-clamping on neonatal outcomes and iron status at four months: a randomized controlled trial. *BMJ*. 2011;343:d7157.

McDonald SJ, Middleton P. Effect of timing of umbilical cord-clamping of term infants on maternal and neonatal outcomes. *Cochrane Database Syst Rev.* 2008;2:CD004074.

Ouch!

What's more painful: childbirth or having your leg chopped off?

Lowe NK. The nature of labor pain. *Am J Obstet Gynecol.* 2002 May;186(5):S16–24.

Lally JE, Murtagh MJ, Macphail S, Thomson R. More in hope than expectation: a systematic review of women's expectations and experience of pain relief in labor. *BMC Med.* 2008 Mar;6, art. 7.

Melzack R, Taenzer P, Feldman P, Kinch RA. Labor is still painful after prepared childbirth training. *Can Med Assoc J.* 1981 Aug 15;125:357.

Do hormones block the pain of labor?

Brownridge P. The nature and consequences of childbirth pain. *Eur J Obstetr Gynecol Reprod Biol.* 1995 May;59:S9–15.

Ohel I, Walfisch A, Shitenberg D, Sheiner E, Hallak M. A rise in pain threshold during labor: a prospective clinical trial. *Pain.* 2007 Nov;132 (suppl. 1):S104–8.

Bajaj P, Bajaj P, Madsen H, Møller M, Arendt-Nielsen L. Antenatal women with or without pelvic pain can be characterized by generalized or segmental hypoalgesia in late pregnancy. *J Pain.* 2002 Dec;3(6):451–60.

Why do women come back for more?

Waldenström U, Schytt E. A longitudinal study of women's memory of labor pain. *BJOG.* 2009 Mar;116(4):577–83.

Heinrichs M, Meinlschmidt G, Wippich W, Ehlert U, Hellhammer DH. Selective amnesic effects of oxytocin on human memory. *Physiol Behav.* 2004 Oct;83(1):31–8.

Can hypnosis or alternative therapies reduce labor pain?

Jones L, Othman M, Dowswell T, Alfirevic Z, Gates S, Newburn M, Jordan S, Lavender T, Neilson JP. Pain management for women in labour: an overview of systematic reviews. *Cochrane Database Syst Rev.* 2012;3:CD009234.

Cluett ER, Burns E. Immersion in water in labor and birth. *Cochrane Database Syst Rev.* 2009;2:CD000111.

Cho SH, Lee H, Ernst E. Acupuncture for pain relief in labor: a systematic review and meta-analysis. *BJOG*. 2010 Jul;117(8):907–20.

Smith CA, Collins CT, Crowther CA. Aromatherapy for pain management in labor *Cochrane Database Syst Rev.* 2011 Jul;7:CD009215.

Does an epidural make a C-section more likely?

Anim-Somuah M, Smyth RMD, Jones L. Epidural versus non-epidural or no analgesia in labor. *Cochrane Database Syst Rev.* 2011;12:CD000331.

Jones L, Othman M, Dowswell T, Alfirevic Z, Gates S, Newburn M, Jordan S, Lavender T, Neilson JP. Pain management for women in labour: an overview of systematic reviews. *Cochrane Database Syst Rev.* 2012;3:CD009234.

Pennell A, Salo-Coombs V, Herring A, Spielman F, Fecho K. Anesthesia and analgesia-related preferences and outcomes of women who have birth plans. *J Midwifery Womens Health*. 2011 Jul-Aug;56(4):376–81.

Henderson K, Shirgaonkar A, Vipond A, Easaw B. Labour analgesia and the baby: good news is no news. *Int J Obstetr Anesth*. 2011;20(1):38–50.

All About Epidural. Epidural and instrumental delivery (forceps and vacuum). Available from: http://www.allaboutepidural.com/epidural-and-instrumental-delivery.

Christianson LM, Bovbjerg VE, McDavitt EC, Hullfish KL. Risk factors for perineal injury during delivery. *Am J Obstet Gynecol*. 2003 Jul;189(1):255–60.

Do gas and air or Demerol relieve pain?

Henderson K, Shirgaonkar A, Vipond A, Easaw B. Labour analgesia and the baby: good news is no news. *Int J Obstetr Anesth*. 2011;20(1):38–50.

Jones L, Othman M, Dowswell T, Alfirevic Z, Gates S, Newburn M, Jordan S, Lavender T, Neilson JP. Pain management for women in labour: an overview of systematic reviews. *Cochrane Database Syst Rev.* 2012;3:CD009234.

Tsui MH, Ngan Kee WD, Ng FF, Lau TK. A double-blinded randomised placebo-controlled study of intramuscular pethidine for pain relief in the first stage of labor. *BJOG*. 2004 Jul;111(7):648–55.

The Post-Pregnancy Body

What causes the baby blues?

Sacher J, Wilson AA, Houle S, Rusjan P, Hassan S, Bloomfield PM, Stewart DE, Meyer JH. Elevated brain monoamine oxidase A binding in the early postpartum period. *Arch Gen Psychiatry*. 2010 May;67(5):468.

McQueen K, Montgomery P, Lappan-Gracon S, Evans M, Hunter J. Evidence-based recommendations for depressive symptoms in postpartum women. *J Obstetr Gynecol Neonatal Nurs.* 2008 Mar 11;37(2):127.

Why can't I poop?

Henderson C, Macdonald S, eds. *Mayes' midwifery: a textbook for midwives.* 13th ed. London: Baillière Tindall; 2004.

St. Mark's Hospital, London. Constipation. [Patient information leaflet.]

How do I know if my stitches are okay?

Perineal care. *Clinical Evidence* (online). 2010 Mar.

Johnson A, Thakar R, Sultan AH. Obstetric perineal wound infection: is there under-reporting? *Br J Nurs.* 2012 Mar 8;21(5):S28.

Calvert S, Fleming V. Minimizing postpartum pain: a review of research pertaining to perineal care in childbearing women. *J Adv Nurs.* 2000 Aug;32(2):407.

East CE, Begg L, Henshall NE, Marchant PR, Wallace K. Local cooling for relieving pain from perineal trauma sustained during childbirth. *Cochrane Database Syst Rev.* 2012 May;5:CD006304.

Is it normal to be turned off by sex after birth?

LaMarre AK, Paterson LQ, Gorzalka BB. Breastfeeding and postpartum maternal sexual functioning: A review. *CJHS* 2003. Fall/Winter 12 (3–4): 151–168.

Is there anything I can do to stop my breasts sagging after breast-feeding?

Pisacane A, Continisio P; Italian Work Group on Breastfeeding. Breast-feeding and perceived changes in the appearance of the breasts: a retrospective study. *Acta Pediatr.* 2004;93(10):1346–8.

Rinker B, Veneracion M, Walsh CP. Breast ptosis: causes and cure. *Ann Plast Surg.* 2010 May;64(5):579–84.

The female breast: structure and changes in pregnancy and lactation. Midwives Information and Resource Service Practice Development. 2011 Jun.

Do women who breast-feed really lose their baby weight faster than those who bottle-feed?

Dewey KG. Impact of breastfeeding on maternal nutritional status. *Adv Exp Med Biol.* 2004;554:91–100.

Lovelady C. Balancing exercise and food intake with lactation to promote postpartum weight loss. *Proc Nutr Soc.* 2011 May;70(2):181–4.

Do cells from my baby live on in my body after birth?

Fugazzola L, Cirello V, Beck-Peccoz P. Fetal microchimerism as an explanation of disease. *Nat Rev Endocrinol*. 2011 Feb;7:89–97.

Tan XW, Liao H, Sun L, Okabe M, Xiao ZC, Dawe GS. Fetal microchimerism in the maternal mouse brain: a novel population of fetal progenitor or stem cells able to cross the blood-brain barrier? *Stem Cells*. 2005 Nov;23(10):1443–52.

Boyon C, Collinet P, Boulanger L, Rubod C, Lucot JP, Vinatier D. Fetal microchimerism: benevolence or malevolence for the mother? *Eur J Obstet Gynecol Reprod Biol*. 2011 Oct;158(2):148–52.

Gammill HS, Adams Waldorf KM, Aydelotte TM, Lucas J, Leisenring WM, Lambert NC, Nelson JL. Pregnancy, microchimerism and the maternal grandmother. *PLoS One*. 2011;6(8): e24101.

Three: Babies
Portrait of a Newborn

Does birth distress the baby?

Bergqvist LL, Katz-Salamon M, Hertegård S, Anand KJ, Lagercrantz H. Mode of delivery modulates physiological and behavioral responses to neonatal pain. *J Perinatol*. 2009 Jan;29:4–50.

Mazzuca M, Minlebaev M, Shakirzyanova A, Tyzio R, Taccola G, Janackova S, Gataullina S, Ben-Ari Y, Giniatullin R, Khazipov R. Newborn analgesia mediated by oxytocin during delivery. *Front Cell Neurosci*. 2011 Apr;5:3.

Khazipov R, Tyzio R, Ben-Ari Y. Effects of oxytocin on GABA signalling in the foetal brain during delivery. *Prog Brain Res*. 2008;170:243–57.

Why do newborns look like their dads?

Christenfeld NJ, Hill EA. Whose baby are you? *Nature*. 1995 Dec 14;378(6558):669.

Bellis MA, Hughes K, Hughes S, Ashton JR. Measuring paternal discrepancy and its public health consequences. *J Epidemiol Community Health*. 2005;59:749–54.

French RM, Brédart S, Huart J, Labiouse CL. The resemblance of one-year-old infants to their fathers: refuting Christenfeld and Hill (1995). In: Gleitman L, Joshi AK, ed. *Proceedings of the twenty-second annual conference of the Cognitive Science Society*. Mahwah, NJ: Erlbaum; 2000.

What do newborns know?

Slater A, Lewis M, eds. *Introduction to infant development*. 2nd ed. Oxford: Oxford University Press; 2007.

DeCasper AJ, Fifer WP. Of human bonding: newborns prefer their mothers' voices. *Science*. 1980;208(4448):1174–6.

Porter RH. The biological significance of skin-to-skin contact and maternal odors. *Acta Paediatr*. 2004;93:1560–2.

Bushnell IWR, Sai F, Mullin JT. Neonatal recognition of the mother's face. *Br J Devel Psychol*. 1989;7(1):3–15.

Meltzoff AN, Moore MK. Newborn infants imitate adult facial gestures. *Child Dev*.1983 Jun;54(3):702–9.

Batki A, Baron-Cohen S, Wheelwright S, Connellan J, Ahluwalia J. Is there an innate gaze module? Evidence from human neonates. *Infant Behav Devel*. 2000 Feb;23(2):223–9.

Farroni T. The perception of facial expressions in newborns. *Eur J Dev Psychol*. 2007 Mar;4(1):2–13.

Izard V, Sann C, Spelke ES, Streri A. Newborn infants perceive abstract numbers. *Proc Natl Acad Sci*. 2009 Jun 23;106(25):10382–5.

Slater A, Lewis M, eds. *Introduction to infant development*. 2nd ed. Oxford: Oxford University Press; 2007.

Mehler J, Jusczyk P, Lambertz G, Halsted N, Bertoncini J, Amiel-Tison C. A precursor of language acquisition in young infants. *Cognition*. 1988;29:143–78.

Mastropieri D, Turkewitz G. Prenatal experience and neonatal responsiveness to vocal expressions of emotion. *Dev Psychobiol*. 1999 Nov;35(3):204–14.

Mampe B, Friederici AD, Christophe A, Wermke K. Newborns' cry melody is shaped by their native language. *Curr Biol*. 2009 Dec 15;19(23):1994–7.

Dondi M, Simion F, Caltran G. Can newborns discriminate between their own cry and the cry of another newborn infant? *Dev Psychol*. 1999;35(2):418–26.

Gopnik A, Meltzoff A, Kuhl P. *How babies think*. London: Phoenix; 1999.

Winkler I, Háden GP, Ladinig O, Sziller I, Honing H. Newborn infants detect the beat in music. *Proc Natl Acad Sci U S A*. 2009 Feb 17;106(7):2468–71.

How much can newborns see?

Norcia AM, Tyler CW, Hamer RD. Development of contrast sensitivity in the human infant. *Vision Res*. 1990;30(10):1475–86.

Allen D, Banks MS, Norcia AM. Does chromatic sensitivity develop more slowly than luminance sensitivity? *Vision Res*. 1993;33(17):2553–62.

How do babies go from breathing nothing to breathing air?

Henderson C, Macdonald S, eds. *Mayes' midwifery: a textbook for midwives*. 13th ed. London: Baillière Tindall; 2004.

Adamson SL. Regulation of breathing at birth. *J Dev Physiol.* 1991 Jan;15(1):45–52.

Togari H, Sobajima H, Suzuki S. Oxygen and reduced umbilical blood flow trigger the first breath of human neonates. *Acta Paediatr.* 1992;34:660–2.

Mercer JS, Skovgaard RL. Neonatal transitional physiology: a new paradigm. *J Perinat Neonatal Nurs.* 2002;15(4):56–75.

Why do newborn babies smell so good?

Porter RH. Olfaction and human kin recognition. *Genetica.* 1999;104:259–63.

Fleming AS, Steiner M, Corter C. Cortisol, hedonics, and maternal responsiveness in human mothers. *Horm Behav.* 1997 Oct;32(2):85–98.

Porter RH, Winberg J. Unique salience of maternal breast odors for newborn infants. *Neurosci Biobehav Rev.* 1999 Jan;23(3):439–49.

Does skin-to-skin contact really soothe my baby?

Moore ER, Anderson GC, Bergman N. Early skin-to-skin contact for mothers and their healthy newborn infants. *Cochrane Database Syst Rev.* 2007(3): CD003519.

Winberg J. Mother and newborn baby: mutual regulation of physiology and behavior—a selective review. *Dev Psychobiol.* 2005;47(3):217–229.

Matthiesen AS, Ransjö-Arvidson AB, Nissen E, Uvnäs-Moberg K. Postpartum maternal oxytocin release by newborns: effects of infant hand massage and sucking. *Birth.* 2001;28(1):13–19.

Erlandsson K, Dsilna A, Fagerberg I, Christensson K. Skin-to-skin care with the father after cesarean birth and its effect on newborn crying and prefeeding behavior. *Birth.* 2007;34(2):105–114.

How do newborns know to seek the nipple for food?

Varendi H, Porter RH. Breast odour as the only maternal stimulus elicits crawling towards the odor source. *Acta Paediatr.* 2001 Apr;90(4):372–5.

Porter RH. The biological significance of skin-to-skin contact and maternal odors. *Acta Paediatr.* 2004 Dec;93(12):1560–62.

Doucet S, Soussignan R, Sagot P, Schaal B. The secretion of areolar (Montgomery's) glands from lactating women elicits selective, unconditional responses in neonates. *PLoS ONE.* 2009;4(10):e7579.

Doucet S, Soussignan R, Sagot P, Schaal B. An overlooked aspect of the human breast: areolar glands in relation with breast-feeding pattern, neonatal weight gain, and the dynamics of lactation. *Early Hum Dev.* 2012 Feb;88(2):119–28.

Spencer NA, McClintock MK, Sellergren SA, Bullivant S, Jacob S, Mennella JA. Social chemosignals from breastfeeding women increase sexual motivation. *Horm Behav.* 2004 Sep;46:362–70.

What causes the Moro or "startle" reflex?

Berk LE. Infancy: early learning, motor skills, and perceptual capacity. In: Berk LE, *Child Development*, 7th ed. Boston: Pearson/Allyn and Bacon; 2006.

Futagi Y, Toribe Y, Suzuki Y. The grasp reflex and Moro reflex in infants: hierarchy of primitive reflex responses. *Int J Pediatr*. 2012. DOI: 10.1155/2012/191562.

Baby Bodies

Are baby growth charts accurate?

Wright CM, Williams AF, Elliman D, Bedford H, Birks E, Butler G, Sachs M, Moy RJ, Cole TJ. Using the new UK-WHO growth charts. *BMJ*. 2010;340:c1140.

Ziegler EE, Nelson SE. The WHO growth standards: strengths and limitations. *Curr Opin Clin Nutr Metab Care*. 2012 May;15(3):298–302.

Do big babies grow into big adults?

Sørensen HT, Sabroe S, Rothman KJ, Gillman M, Steffensen FH, Fischer P, Sørensen TI. Birth weight and length as predictors for adult height. *Am J Epidemiol*. 1999;149(8):726–9.

Eide MG, Øyen N, Skjaerven R, Nilsen ST, Bjerkedal T, Tell GS. Size at birth and gestational age as predictors of adult height and weight. *Epidemiol*. 2005 Mar, 16(2):175–81.

Why don't babies have moles?

American Academy of Dermatology. Moles in children: what parents should know. Fact sheet. Available from: http://www.skincarephysicians.com/skincancernet/moles_children.html.

Wachsmuth RC, Turner F, Barrett JH, Gaut R, Randerson-Moor JA, Bishop DT, Bishop JA. The effect of sun exposure in determining nevus density in UK adolescent twins. *J Invest Dermatol*. 2005;124:56–62.

What causes colic?

Douglas P, Hill P. Managing infants who cry excessively in the first few months of life. *BMJ*. 2011 Dec;343:d7772.

Vandenplas Y, Koletzko S, Isolauri E, Hill D, Oranje AP, Brueton M, Staiano A, Dupont C. Guidelines for the diagnosis and management of cow's milk protein allergy in infants. *Arch Dis Child*. 2007;92:902–8.

Miller-Loncar C, Bigsby R, High P, Wallach M, Lester B. Infant colic and feeding difficulties. *Arch Dis Child*. 2004;89:908–12.

Sherman PM, Hassall E, Fagundes-Neto U, Gold BD, Kato S, Koletzko S, Orenstein S, Rudolph C, Vakil N, Vandenplas Y. A global, evidence-based consensus on the definition of gastroesophageal reflux disease in the pediatric population. *Am J Gastroenterol*. 2009;104:1278–95.

Savino F. Focus on infantile colic. *Acta Paediatr*. 2007 Sep;96(9):1259–64.

Winter HS. Patient information: acid reflux (gastroesophageal reflux) in infants (beyond the basics). Up to Date (website), Wolters Kluwer Health. Available from: http://www.uptodate.com/contents/acid-reflux-gastroesophageal-reflux-in-infants-beyond-the-basics.

Colic in babies: An NCT evidence-based briefing. *New Digest*. 2008 Apr.

What is the best way to settle a crying baby?

Evanoo G. Infant crying: a clinical conundrum. *J Pediatr Health Care*. 2007;21:333–8.

van Sleuwen BE, Engelberts AC, Boere-Boonekamp MM, Kuis W, Schulpen TW, L'Hoir MP. Swaddling: a systematic review. *Pediatrics*. 2007 Oct 1;120(4):e1097–e1106.

van Sleuwen BE, L'hoir MP, Engelberts AC, Busschers WB, Westers P, Blom MA, Schulpen TW, Kuis W. Comparison of behavior modification with and without swaddling as interventions for excessive crying. *J Pediatr*. 2006 Oct;149(4):512–17, e2.

Ernst E. Chiropractic spinal manipulation for infant colic: a systematic review of randomised clinical trials. *Int J Clin Pract*. 2009 Sep;63(9):1351–3.

St. James-Roberts I, Peachey E. Distinguishing infant prolonged crying from sleep-waking problems. *Arch Dis Child*. 2011 Apr;96(4):340–4.

Douglas P, Hill P. Managing infants who cry excessively in the first few months of life. *BMJ*. 2011;343:d7772.

Underdown A, Barlow J, Chung V, Stewart-Brown S. Massage intervention for promoting mental and physical health in infants aged under six months. *Cochrane Database Syst Rev*. 2006;4:CD005038.

Why do some belly buttons become "outies"?

Sinkkonen A. Umbilicus as a fitness signal in humans. *FASEB J*. 2009;23(1):10–12.

Cavale N, Butler PE. In search of the ideal female umbilicus. *Plast Reconstr Surg*. 2008;105(1):389–92.

Do babies heal faster than adults?

Bermudez DM, Canning DA, Liechty KW. Age and pro-inflammatory cytokine production: wound-healing implications for scar-formation and the timing of genital surgery in boys. *J Pediatr Urol*. 2011 Jun;7(3):324–31.

Porrello ER, Mahmoud AI, Simpson E, Hill JA, Richardson JA, Olson EN, Sadek HA. Transient regenerative potential of the neonatal mouse heart. *Science*. 2011 Feb 25;331(6020):1078–80.

Why do babies gnaw on things even before they start teething?

Wake M, Hesketh K, Lucas J. Teething and tooth eruption in infants: a cohort study. *Pediatrics*. 2000 Dec;106(6):1374–9.

Ramos-Jorge J, Pordeus IA, Ramos-Jorge ML, Paiva SM. Prospective longitudinal study of signs and symptoms associated with primary tooth eruption. *Pediatrics*. 2011 Sep;128(3):e1–e6.

Why is baby hair a different color from adult hair, and why do babies lose their hair?

Furdon SA, Clark DA. Scalp hair characteristics in the newborn infant: scalp hair examination. *Adv Neonatal Care*. 2003;3(6):286–96.

Barth JH. Normal hair growth in children. *Pediatr Dermatol*. 1987;4(3):n173–84.

Fletcher MA. Head and neck region. In: Fletcher MA, *Physical Diagnosis in Neonatology*. Philadelphia: Lippincott-Raven; 1998.

Can newborns sweat?

Harpin VA, Rutter N. Sweating in preterm babies. *J Pediatr*. 1982 Apr;100(4):614–19.

Are pacifiers good or bad for babies?

Hauck FR, Omojokun OO, Siadaty MS. Do pacifiers reduce the risk of sudden infant death syndrome? A meta-analysis. *Pediatrics*. 2005 Nov;116(5):e716–23.

Sexton S, Natale R. Risks and benefits of pacifiers. *Am Fam Physician*. 2009 Apr 15;79(8):681–5.

Sleep

Can babies tell the difference between night and day?

Rivkees SA. Developing circadian rhythmicity in infants. *Pediatrics*. 2003 Aug 1;112(2):373–81.

Are a baby's sleep patterns inherited?

Mongrain V, Paquet J, Dumont M. Contribution of the photoperiod at birth to the association between season of birth and diurnal preference. *Neurosci Lett.* 2006;406:113–16.

Brescianini S, Volzone A, Fagnani C, Patriarca V, Grimaldi V, Lanni R, Serino L, Mastroiacovo P, Stazi MA. Genetic and environmental factors shape infant sleep patterns: a study of eighteen-month-old twins. *Pediatrics.* 2011 May;127(5):e1296–1302.

St. James-Roberts I, Plewis I. Individual differences, daily fluctuations, and developmental changes in amounts of infant waking, fussing, crying, feeding, and sleeping. *Child Devel.* 1996 Oct;67(5):2527–40.

How can I get my baby to sleep through the night?

What influences baby-sleeping behavior at night? A review of evidence. *New Digest.* 2008 Apr.

Pinilla T, Birch LL. Help me make it through the night: behavioral entrainment of breast-fed infants' sleep patterns. *Pediatrics.* 1993 Feb;91(2):436–44.

St James-Roberts I, Sleep J, Morris S, Owen C, Gillham P. Use of a behavioural programme in the first three months to prevent infant crying and sleeping problems. *J Paediatr Child Health.* 2001 Jun;37(3):289–97.

Is co-sleeping good or bad for my baby?

Ramos KD, Youngclarke DM. Parenting advice books about child sleep: co-sleeping and crying it out. *Sleep.* 2006 Dec;29(12):1616–23.

Ball H. Research overview: bed-sharing and co-sleeping. *New Digest.* 2009 Oct.

Okami P, Weisner T, Olmstead R. Outcome correlates of parent-child bedsharing: an eighteen-year longitudinal study. *J Dev Behav Pediatr.* 2002 Aug;23(4):244–53.

Kelmanson IA. Parent-infant bed sharing and behavioural features in 2–4-month-old infants. *Early Child Dev Care.* 1999;149(1):1–9.

Crawford CJ. Parenting practices in the Basque country: implications of infant and childhood sleeping location for personality development. *Ethos.* 1994;22:42–82.

McKenna JJ, McDade T. Why babies should never sleep alone: a review of the co-sleeping controversy in relation to SIDS, bedsharing and breast-feeding. *Paedr Respir Rev.* 2005;6:134–52.

Thoman EB. Co-sleeping, an ancient practice: issues of the past and present, and possibilities for the future. *Sleep Med Rev.* 2006;10:407–17.

Will leaving my baby to cry cause any long-term damage?

Mindell JA, Kuhn B, Lewin DS, Meltzer LJ, Sadeh A; American Academy of Sleep Medicine. Behavioral treatment of bedtime problems and night wakings in infants and young children. *Sleep*. 2006 Oct;29(10):1263–76.

Ramos KD, Youngclarke DM. Parenting advice books about child sleep: co-sleeping and crying it out. *Sleep*. 2006 Dec;29(12):1616–23.

Middlemiss W, Granger DA, Goldberg WA, Nathans L. Asynchrony of mother-infant hypothalamic-pituitary-adrenal axis activity following extinction of infant crying responses induced during the transition to sleep. *Early Hum Dev.* 2012 Apr;88:227–32.

Price AM, Wake M, Ukoumunne OC, Hiscock H. Five-year follow-up of harms and benefits of behavioral infant sleep intervention: randomized trial. *Pediatrics*. 2012 Sep;DOI:10.1542/peds.2011–3467.

What's more effective: introducing strict routines or immediately responding to my baby's demands?

St. James-Roberts I, Alvarez M, Csipke E, Abramsky T, Goodwin J, Sorgenfrei E. Infant crying and sleeping in London, Copenhagen and when parents adopt a "proximal" form of care. *Pediatrics*. 2006 Jun;117(6):e1146–e1155.

The White Stuff

How does breast-feeding work?

Geddes D. Infant gastric physiology—ultrasound studies of the term and preterm infants. Presentation at Seventh International Breast-feeding and Lactation Symposium, Vienna, Austria, 2012 Apr 20–21.

Should I feed on demand or wait three to four hours between feeds?

Kent JC. How breast-feeding works. *J Midwifery Womens Health*. 2007 Nov-Dec;52(6):564–70.

Kent JC, Mitoulas LR, Cregan MD, Ramsay DT, Doherty DA, Hartmann PE. Volume and frequency of breastfeedings and fat content of breast milk throughout the day. *Pediatrics*. 2006 Mar 1;117(3):e387–95.

Is breast really best for babies?

Kramer MS. "Breast is best": the evidence. *Early Hum Dev.* 2010 Nov;86:729–32.

American Academy of Pediatrics. Breastfeeding and the use of human milk. *Pediatrics*. 2012;129:e827.

Krebs NF. Infant feeding matters. *J Pediatr.* 2011;159(2):175–6.

Pearson H. Children of the 90s: coming of age. *Nature.* 2012 Apr 11;484(7393): 155–8.

How long do I need to breast-feed in order for my baby to reap the benefits?

American Academy of Pediatrics. Breastfeeding and the use of human milk. *Pediatrics.* 2012;129:e827.

Holmes AV, Auinger P, Howard CR. Combination feeding of breast milk and formula: evidence for shorter breast-feeding duration from the National Health and Nutrition Examination Survey. *J Pediatr.* 2011;159(2):186–90.

Could combining breast- and formula-feeding offer babies the best of both worlds?

Holmes AV, Auinger P, Howard CR. Combination feeding of breast milk and formula: evidence for shorter breast-feeding duration from the National Health and Nutrition Examination Survey. *J Pediatr.* 2011;159(2):186–90.

What is in formula milk, and why does it taste fishy?

Dodds R. Choosing a formula—what is the evidence for different milks and added ingredients? *New Digest.* 2010 Jul.

O'Connor NR. Infant formula. *Am Fam Physician.* 2009 Apr 1;79(7):565–70.

Martinez JA. Infant formulas. *Pediatr Rev.* 2011;32(5):179–89.

Does "nipple confusion" really exist?

Holmes AV, Auinger P, Howard CR. Combination feeding of breast milk and formula: evidence for shorter breast-feeding duration from the National Health and Nutrition Examination Survey. *J Pediatr.* 2011;159(2):186–90.

Al-Sahab B, Feldman M, Macpherson A, Ohlsson A, Tamim H. Which method of breastfeeding supplementation is best? The beliefs and practices of paediatricians and nurses. *Paediatr Child Health.* 2010 Sep;15(7):427–31.

Flint A, New K, Davies MW. Cup feeding versus other forms of supplemental enteral feeding for newborn infants unable to fully breast-feed. *Cochrane Database Syst Rev.* 2007 Apr;2:CD005092.

O'Connor NR, Tanabe KO, Siadaty MS, Hauck FR. Pacifiers and breastfeeding: a systematic review. *Arch Pediatr Adolesc Med.* 2009;163(4):378–82.

Jaafar SH, Jahanfar S, Angolkar M, Ho JJ. Pacifier use versus no pacifier use in breast-feeding term infants for increasing duration of breast-feeding. *Cochrane Database Syst Rev.* 2011;3:CD007202.

Does what I eat change the flavor of my milk?

Hausner H, Bredie WL, Mølgaard C, Petersen MA, Møller P. Differential transfer of dietary flavor compounds into human breast milk. *Physiol Behav*. 2008 Sep 3;95(1–2):118–24.

How much alcohol gets into breast milk?

Kesäniemi YA. Ethanol and acetaldehyde in the milk and peripheral blood of lactating women after ethanol administration. *J Obstet Gynaecol Br Commonwealth*. 1974 Jan;81:84–6.

Lawton ME. Alcohol in breast milk. *Aust N Z J Obstet Gynaecol*. 1985 Feb;25:71–3.

Mennella JA, Gerrish CJ. Effects of exposure to alcohol in mother's milk on infant sleep. *Pediatrics*. 1998 May 1;101(5):e2.

Bowen A, Tumback L. Alcohol and breastfeeding: dispelling the myths and promoting the evidence. *Nurs Womens Health*. 2011 Dec-Jan;14(6):454–61.

Is morning breast milk any different from evening breast milk?

Sánchez CL, Cubero J, Sánchez J, Chanclón B, Rivero M, Rodríguez AB, Barriga C. The possible role of human milk nucleotides as sleep inducers. *Nutr Neurosci*. 2009 Feb;12(1):2–8.

Blyton DM, Sullivan CE, Edwards N. Lactation is associated with an increase in slow-wave sleep in women. *J Sleep Res*. 2002 Dec.;11(4):297–303.

Can men lactate?

Kulski JK, Hartmann PE, Gutteridge DH. Composition of breast fluid of a man with galactorrhea and hyperprolactinaemia. *J Clin Endocrinol Metab*. 1981 Mar 1;52(3):581–2.

Weaning

When should I wean my baby onto solid foods?

Mehta KC, Specker BL, Bartholmey S, Giddens J, Ho ML. Trial on timing of introduction to solids and food type on infant growth. *Pediatrics*. 1998 Sep;102:569–73.

NCT evidence-based briefing: when can babies start on solids? *New Digest*. 2002 Oct:22–5.

Morgan JB, Lucas A, Fewtrell MS. Does weaning influence growth and health up to eighteen months? *Arch Dis Child*. 2004 Aug;89:728–33.

UK Scientific Advisory Committee on Nutrition Subgroup on Maternal and Child Nutrition (SMCN). Paper for discussion: introduction of solid foods. 2003 Sep 29.

Zutavern A, Brockow I, Schaaf B, von Berg A, Diez U, Borte M, Kraemer U, Herbarth O, Behrendt H, Wichmann HE, Heinrich J; LISA Study Group. Timing of solid food introduction in relation to eczema, asthma, allergic rhinitis, and food and inhalant sensitization at the age of six years: results from the Prospective Birth Cohort Study LISA. *Pediatrics*. 2008 Jan 1;121(1):e44–52.

Huh SY, Rifas-Shiman SL, Taveras EM, Oken E, Gillman MW. Timing of solid food introduction and risk of obesity in preschool-aged children. *Pediatrics*. 2011 Mar 1;127(3):e544–e551.

ESPGHAN Committee on Nutrition, Agostoni C, Braegger C, Decsi T, Kolacek S, Koletzko B, Michaelsen KF, Mihatsch W, Moreno LA, Puntis J, Shamir R, Szajewska H, Turck D, van Goudoever J. Complementary feeding: a commentary by the ESPGHAN Committee on Nutrition. *J Pediatr Gastroenterol Nutr*. 2008 Jan;46(1):99–110.

How do I get my baby to like vegetables?

Mennella JA, Nicklaus S, Jagolino AL, Yourshaw LM. Variety is the spice of life: strategies for promoting fruit and vegetable acceptance during infancy. *Physiol Behav*. 2008 Apr 22;94(1):29–38.

Capaldi ED, Privitera GJ. Decreasing dislike for sour and bitter in children and adults. *Appetite*. 2008 Jan;50(1):139–45.

Heath P, Houston-Price C, Kennedy OB. Increasing food familiarity without the tears. A role for visual exposure? *Appetite*. 2011 Dec;57(3):832–8.

Is there any evidence for baby-led weaning being better than parent-led weaning?

Townsend E, Pitchford NJ. Baby knows best? The impact of weaning style on food preferences and body mass index in early childhood in a case-controlled sample. *BMJ Open*. 2012;2:e000298.

Wright CM, Cameron K, Tsiaka M, Parkinson KN. Is baby-led weaning feasible? When do babies first reach out for and eat finger foods? *Matern Child Nutr*. 2011 Jan;7(1):27–33.

Should I force my baby to eat?

Brown A, Lee M. Maternal control of child feeding during the weaning period: differences between mothers following a baby-led or standard weaning approach. *Matern Child Health J*. 2011 Nov;15(8):1265–71.

Farrow C, Blissett J. Does maternal control during feeding moderate early infant weight gain? *Pediatrics*. 2006 Aug 1;118(2):e293–e298.

How many calories does a baby need?

Butte NF. Energy requirements of infants. *Public Health Nutr*. 2005;8(7A):953–67.

Should I avoid feeding my baby nuts or eggs to protect it against allergies?

ESPGHAN Committee on Nutrition, Agostoni C, Braegger C, Decsi T, Kolacek S, Koletzko B, Michaelsen KF, Mihatsch W, Moreno LA, Puntis J, Shamir R, Szajewska H, Turck D, van Goudoever J. Complementary feeding: a commentary by the ESPGHAN Committee on Nutrition. *J Pediatr Gastroenterol Nutr*. 2008 Jan;46(1):99–110.

Greer FR, Sicherer SH, Burks AW; American Academy of Pediatrics Committee on Nutrition; American Academy of Pediatrics Section on Allergy and Immunology. Effects of early nutritional interventions on the development of atopic disease in infants and children: the role of maternal dietary restriction, breastfeeding, timing of introduction of complementary foods, and hydrolyzed formulas. *Pediatrics*. 2008 Jan 1;121(1):183–91.

The Brown Stuff

Are reusable diapers really greener than disposables?

UK Environment Agency. An updated lifecycle assessment study for disposable and reusable nappies. Science Report SC010018/SR 2. 2008 Oct.

Baer EL, Davies MW, Easterbrook K. Disposable nappies for preventing napkin dermatitis in infants. *Cochrane Database Syst Rev*. 2006;3:CD004262.

Why does baby poop smell like mustard?

Jiang T, Suarez FL, Levitt MD, Nelson SE, Ziegler EE. Gas production by feces of infants. *J Pediatr Gastroenterol Nutr*. 2001 May;32:534–41.

Case TI. My baby doesn't smell as bad as yours: the plasticity of disgust. *Evolution and Hum Behav*. 2006 Sep;27(5):357–65.

Baby Brains

Is the temperament of a newborn carried through into childhood and beyond?

Rothbart MK, Ahadi SA, Evans DE. Temperament and personality: origins and outcomes. *J Pers Soc Psychol*. 2000;78(1):122–35.

McAdams DP, Olson BD. Personality development: continuity and change over the life course. *Annu Rev Psychol.* 2010 Jan;61:517–42.

Saudino KJ. Behavioral genetics and child temperament. *J Dev Behav Pediatr.* 2005 Jun;26(3):214–23.

Bohlin G, Hagekull B. Socio-emotional development: from infancy to young adulthood. *Scand J Psychol.* 2009 Dec;50(6):592–601.

Fox NA. Does infancy matter? Predicting social behavior from infant temperament. *Infant Behav Dev.* 1999;22(4):445–55.

When do babies develop a sense of themselves as individuals?

Slater A, Lewis M, eds. *Introduction to infant development.* 2nd ed. Oxford: Oxford University Press; 2007.

Can parents modify their baby's personality traits?

Rothbart MK. Temperament and personality: origins and outcomes. *J Pers Soc Psychol.* 2000;78(1):122–35.

McAdams DP, Olson BD. Personality development: continuity and change over the life course. *Ann Rev Psychol.* 2010 Jan;61:517–42.

van den Boom DC. The influence of temperament and mothering on attachment and exploration: an experimental manipulation of sensitive responsiveness among lower-class mothers with irritable infants. *Child Dev.* 1994 Oct;65(5):1457–77.

Chen X, DeSouza AT, Chen H, Wang L. Reticent behavior and experiences in peer interactions in Chinese and Canadian children. *Dev Psychol.* 2006 Jul;42(4):656–65.

Does the order of birth influence children's personalities?

Hartshorne JK. How birth order affects your personality. *Scientific American Mind.* 2010 Jan 11.

Kristensen P, Bjerkedal T. Explaining the relation between birth order and intelligence. *Science.* 2007 Jun;316(5832):1717.

Sullaway F. Why siblings are like Darwin's finches: birth order, sibling competition and adaptive divergence within the family. In: Sullaway F, *The evolution of personality and individual differences.* Oxford: Oxford University Press; 2010.

Bouchard TJ Jr, Lykken DT, McGue M, Segal NL, Tellegen A. Sources of human psychological differences: the Minnesota study of twins reared apart. *Science.* 1990 Oct;250(4978):223–8.

Why do twins develop different personalities?

Riese ML. Neonatal temperament in monozygotic and dizygotic twin pairs. *Child Dev.* 1990 Aug;61(4):1230–7.

Spector T. *Identically different: why you can change your genes.* London: Weidenfeld and Nicolson; 2012.

Do babies like some people better than others?

Slater A. Newborn infants prefer attractive faces. *Infant Behav Dev.* 1998;21(2):345–54.

Nagy E. Innate intersubjectivity: newborns' sensitivity to communication disturbance. *Dev Psychol.* 2008 Nov;44(6):1779–84.

Hamlin JK, Wynn K, Bloom P. Social evaluation by preverbal infants. *Nature.* 2007;450:557–9.

How much do babies remember?

Rovee-Collier C. The development of infant memory. *Curr Directions Psychol Sci.* 1999 Jun;8(3):80–5.

Meltzoff AN. What infant memory tells us about infantile amnesia: long-term recall and deferred imitation. *J Exp Child Psychol.* 1995 Jun;59:497–515.

Why don't we remember being babies?

Slater A, Lewis M, eds. *Introduction to infant development.* 2nd ed. Oxford: Oxford University Press; 2007.

Simcock G, Hayne H. Breaking the barrier? Children fail to translate their preverbal memories into language. *Psychol Sci.* 2002 May;13(3):225–31.

Does day care make babies sociable or stressed?

Dettling AC, Parker SW, Lane S, Sebanc A, Gunnar MR. Quality of care and temperament determine changes in cortisol concentrations over the day for young children in childcare. *Psychoneuroendocrinology.* 2000 Nov;25(8):819–36.

Bradley RH, Vandell DL. Child care and the well-being of children. *Arch Pediatr Adolesc Med.* 2007 Jul;161(7):669–76.

U.S. Department of Health and Human Services. *The NICHD study of early childcare and youth development. Findings for children up to age four and a half years.* Washington DC: National Institute of Mental Health; 2006 Jan.

Pluess M, Belsky J. Differential susceptibility to rearing experience: the case of childcare. *J Child Psychol Psychiatry.* 2009 Apr;50(4):396–404.

Are babies born in summer any different from winter babies?

Baxter-Jones A. Born too late to win? *Nature*. 1994 July 21;370:186.

UK Football Association. FA youth development proposals. 2011.

Williams JH. Relative age effect in youth soccer: analysis of the FIFA U17 World Cup competition. *Scand J Med Sci Sports*. 2010;20(3):502–8.

Benson JB. Season of birth and onset of locomotion: theoretical and methodological implications. *Infant Behav Dev*. 1993 Jan-Mar;16(1):69–81.

McGrath JJ, Burne TH, Féron F, Mackay-Sim A, Eyles DW. Developmental vitamin D deficiency and risk of schizophrenia: a ten-year update. *Schizophr Bull*. 2010 Nov;36(6):1073–8.

Motluk A. Born under a bad sign. *New Scientist*. 2007 Jan 27.

Does being born at the start of the school year give you an academic advantage?

Crawford C, Dearden L, Greaves E; Institute for Fiscal Studies. Does when you are born matter? The impact of month of birth on children's cognitive and non-cognitive skills in England. Report to the Nuffield Foundation. 2011 Nov.

Language

When will my baby understand what I'm saying?

Bergelson E, Swingley D. At 6–9 months, human infants know the meanings of many common nouns. *Proc Natl Acad Sci U S A*. 2012 Feb 28;109(9):3253–8.

Why do babies say "Dada" before "Mama"?

Lee SA, Davis B, Macneilage P. Universal production patterns and ambient language influences in babbling: a cross-linguistic study of Korean- and English-learning infants. *J Child Lang*. 2010 Mar;37(2):293–318.

Green JR, Nip ISB. Some organization principles in early speech development. In: Maassen B, van Lieshout P, eds., *Speech motor control: new developments in basic and applied research*. Oxford: Oxford University Press, 2012.

When does baby babble take on meaning?

Holowka S. Left hemisphere cerebral specialization for babies while babbling. *Science*. 2002 Aug 30;297(5586):1515.

Gopnik A, Meltzoff A, Kuhl P. *How babies think*. London: Phoenix; 2001.

Do babies communicate without language?

Goldstein MH, Schwade JA, Bornstein MH. The value of vocalizing: five-month-old infants associate their own noncry vocalizations with responses from caregivers. *Child Dev.* 2009 May-Jun;80(3):636–44.

Liszkowski U, Carpenter M, Tomasello M. Twelve-month-olds communicate helpfully and appropriately for knowledgeable and ignorant partners. *Cognition.* 2008;108:732–39.

Do more physical babies develop language faster than sedentary babies?

Clearfield MW. Learning to walk changes infants' social interactions. *Infant Behav Dev.,* 2011 Feb;34(1):15–25.

Why do women speak to babies in a silly voice?

Kuhl PK, Andruski JE, Chistovich IA, Chistovich LA, Kozhevnikova EV, Ryskina VL, Stolyarova EI, Sundberg U, Lacerda F. Cross-language analysis of phonetic units in language addressed to infants. *Science.* 1997 Aug 1;277:684–6.

Song JY, Demuth K, Morgan J. Effects of the acoustic properties of infant-directed speech on infant word recognition. *J Acoustic Soc Am.* 2010 Jul;128(1):389–400.

Rutherford MD, Przednowek M. Fathers show modifications of infant-directed action similar to that of mothers. *J Exp Child Psychol.* 2012;111:367–78.

When do babies start learning language?

Gopnik A, Meltzoff A, Kuhl P. *How babies think.* London: Phoenix; 2001.

Kuhl PK, Stevens E, Hayashi A, Deguchi T, Kiritani S, Iverson P. Infants show a facilitation effect for native language phonetic perception between six and twelve months. *Dev Sci.* 2006 Mar;9(2):F13–21.

Kuhl PK, Tsao FM, Liu HM. Foreign-language experience in infancy: Effects of short-term exposure and social interaction on phonetic learning. *Proc Natl Acad Sci U S A.* 2003 Jul 22;100(15):9096–9101.

When is the best time to introduce a second language?

Petitto LA, Katerelos M, Levy BG, Gauna K, Tétreault K, Ferraro V. Bilingual signed and spoken language acquisition from birth: implications for the mechanisms underlying early bilingual language acquisition. *J Child Lang.* 2001;28:453–96.

Genesee FH. Early childhood bilingualism: perils and possibilities. *J Appl Res Learning.* 2009 Apr;2:special issue, article 2.

The Next One

Am I likely to become pregnant when breast-feeding?

Gray RH, Campbell OM, Apelo R, Eslami SS, Zacur H, Ramos RM, Gehret JC, Labbok MH. Risk of ovulation during lactation. *Lancet*. 1990;335(8680):25–9.

I had no problem getting pregnant last time, so why am I struggling to conceive now?

Perkins S, Meyers-Thompson J. *Infertility for dummies*. Hoboken, NJ: Wiley; 2007.

Gray RH, Campbell OM, Apelo R, Eslami SS, Zacur H, Ramos RM, Gehret JC, Labbok MH. Risk of ovulation during lactation. *Lancet*. 1990;335(8680):25–9.

Valeggia C, Ellison PT. Interactions between metabolic and reproductive functions in the resumption of postpartum fecundity. *Am J Hum Biol*. 2009;21:559–66.

Why do some women seem to give birth only to boys?

Fukuda M, Fukuda K, Shimizu T, Møller H. Decline in sex ratio at birth after Kobe earthquake. *Hum Reprod*. 1998 Aug;13(8):2321–2.

Catalano R, Bruckner T, Marks AR, Eskenazi B. Exogenous shocks to the human sex ratio: the case of September 11, 2001 in New York City. *Hum Reprod*. 2006 Aug;21(12):3127–31.

Mackenzie CA, Lockridge A, Keith M. Declining sex ratio in a first nation community. *Environ Health Perspect*. 2005 Oct;113(10):1295–8.

Dickinson HO, Parker L, Binks K, Wakeford R, Smith J. The sex ratio of children in relation to paternal preconceptional radiation dose: a study in Cumbria, northern England. *J Epidemiol Community Health*. 1996;50:645–52.

Gellatly C. Trends in population sex ratios may be explained by changes in the frequencies of polymorphic alleles of a sex ratio gene. *Evolutionary Biol*. 2009 Jun;36(2):190–200.

James WH. Offspring sex ratios at birth as markers of paternal endocrine disruption. *Environ Res*. 2006;100:77–85.

Ruckstuhl KE, Colijn GP, Amiot V, Vinish E. Mother's occupation and sex ratio at birth. *BMC Public Health*. 2010 May;10:269.

Magnuson A, Bodin L, Montgomery SM. Father's occupation and sex ratio of offspring. *Scand J Public Health*. 2007;35(5):454–9.

Biggar RJ, Wohlfahrt J, Westergaard T, Melbye M. Sex ratios, family size, and birth order. *Am J Epidemiol*. 1999;150(9):957–62.

Kanazawa S. Beautiful British parents have more daughters. *Reprod Sci.* 2011;18(4):353–8.

Is there anything I can do to influence the gender of my baby?

Cameron EZ, Lemons PR, Bateman PW, Bennett NC. Experimental alteration of litter sex ratios in a mammal. *Proc Biol Sci.* 2008 Feb;275(1632):323–7.

Mathews F, Johnson PJ, Neil A. You are what your mother eats: evidence for maternal preconception diet influencing fetal sex in humans. *Proc Biol Sci.* 2008 Jul;275(1643):1661–8.

Villamor E, Spáren P, Cnattingius S. Interpregnancy weight gain and the male-to-female sex ratio of the second pregnancy: a population-based cohort study. *Fertil Steril.* 2008 May;89(5):1240–4.

Bulik CM, Holle AV, Gendall K, Lie KK, Hoffman E, Mo X, Torgersen L, Reichborn-Kjennerud T. Maternal eating disorders influence sex ratio at birth. *Acta Obstet Gynecol Scand.* 2008;87(9):979–81.

Noorlander AM, Geraedts JP, Melissen JB. Female gender pre-selection by maternal diet in combination with timing of sexual intercourse—a prospective study. *Reprod Biomed Online.* 2010 Dec;21(6):794–802.

Do twins run in families?

Hall JG. Twinning. *Lancet.* 2003;362:735–43.

Painter JN, Willemsen G, Nyholt D, Hoekstra C, Duffy DL, Henders AK, Wallace L, Healey S, Cannon-Albright LA, Skolnick M, Martin NG, Boomsma DI, Montgomery GW. A genome-wide linkage scan for dizygotic twinning in 525 families of mothers of dizygotic twins. *Hum Reprod.* 2010;25(6):1569–80.

Time-lapse recordings reveal why IVF embryos are more likely to develop into twins. *Science News.* 2007 Jul 4.

Glossary

Adrenaline (epinephrine)—A hormone that regulates many of the body's functions, including heart rate and blood pressure, and plays a crucial role in the fight-or-flight response.

Amniotic fluid—The liquid that surrounds and cushions the developing baby in the uterus.

Amniotic sac—The sac containing the baby and amniotic fluid within the uterus. The amniotic sac is what ruptures when a woman's water breaks.

Antenatal—The period before birth (pregnancy). Also known as prenatal.

Apgar score—A score ranging from one to ten that is used to assess the health and appearance of newborn babies at birth.

Attachment—The emotional bond between a baby and its caregiver, which psychologists believe affects the development of personality and the ability to form relationships throughout life.

Bilirubin—The yellow pigment produced during the natural breakdown of red blood cells. Helps give poo its brown color and is responsible for the yellow discoloration of babies with jaundice.

Breech—A breech baby is one lying head-up in the uterus rather than head-down. Babies lying in the breech position when labor begins are more likely to suffer complications during birth, so they are often delivered by C-section instead.

Catecholamines—A group of hormones that are released into the blood during times of physical or emotional stress.

Catheter—A thin plastic tube that is inserted into a vein or the bladder, either to administer fluids or drain the bladder of urine without needing to go to the toilet.

Centers for Disease Control and Prevention (CDC)—The U.S.'s national public health institute.

Cesarean section (C-section)—The surgical procedure in which an incision is made in a woman's abdomen in order to deliver one or more babies.

Classical conditioning—A form of learning in which a stimulus such as food or pain gradually becomes associated with another stimulus.

Cochrane Collaboration—An international nonprofit organization that reviews the results of multiple clinical trials in order to help people make well-informed decisions about health.

Colic—A condition in which an otherwise healthy baby cries for prolonged periods without any obvious reason.

Collagen—The protein found in the skin and connective tissue that provides it with strength and firmness.

Controlled crying—An approach for teaching babies to sleep, which involves putting them to bed awake and leaving them for progressively longer periods if they cry, until they learn to fall asleep by themselves.

Cortisol—A hormone that controls many functions in the body. It is often released during times of stress.

Co-sleeping—Sharing either a bed or a room with your baby.

Diastasis—Separation of the abdominal muscles that occurs during mid- to late pregnancy.

Doppler probe—A handheld device used to detect the baby's heartbeat during pregnancy.

Double-blind study—An experiment in which neither the researchers conducting the study nor the volunteers taking part know which treatment they are receiving.

Dream feed—Involves feeding your baby while it is asleep (usually between ten P.M. and midnight) in the hope of getting a longer stretch of sleep for yourself. *See also* Focal feed.

Embryo—A developing baby is referred to as an embryo until week ten of pregnancy, when it becomes a fetus.

Endometriosis—A medical condition in which cells from the lining of the uterus grow elsewhere in the body.

Endorphins—Also known as "natural painkillers," these brain chemicals are released during pain and strenuous exercise and can promote feelings of well-being.

Epidural—During an epidural, a needle is injected into the small of your back and a small flexible tube inserted, which is then used to deliver painkilling drugs.

Episiotomy—A surgical cut made in the muscular tissue between the vagina and anus to help the baby get out.

Estrogen—The main female sex hormone, which is produced in large amounts during pregnancy and helps the uterus to grow, keeps the lining of the uterus nice and thick, boosts blood circulation and breast development, and helps the baby to grow.

Fibroids—Noncancerous growths in and around the uterus, which can cause pain and heavy bleeding and occasionally impact fertility.

Focal feed—An extra-large breast- or bottle-feed given between ten P.M. and midnight to encourage babies to sleep for longer stretches during the night. *See also* Dream feed.

Fetus—A developing baby is referred to as a fetus from week ten of pregnancy until it is born.

Fetal alcohol syndrome (FAS)—An umbrella term for a range of alcohol-related birth defects.

Forceps—Surgical tongs that can be positioned around a baby's head during delivery and used to help ease it out.

Foremilk—Milk released at the start of a breast feed, which is more watery, lower in fat, and higher in carbohydrates than milk released toward the end of a feed.

Full-term—Babies are considered full-term from thirty-seven weeks of pregnancy and are called premature if they are born before then.

Habituation—A simple form of learning in which a person stops responding to a stimulus such as a sound or picture after being exposed to it lots of times.

Hindmilk—Creamy milk released toward the end of a breast-feed.

Human chorionic gonadotropin—A hormone produced from early pregnancy onward, which can be detected in blood and urine and is what most pregnancy tests look for.

Induced labor—Labor is sometimes started artificially if a baby is overdue or if the mother or baby's health is thought to be at risk.

INSERM (Institut National de la Santé et de la Recherche Médicale)—A French research institution focused on public health.

Instrumental delivery—A birth in which instruments such as forceps or a vacuum device (called a ventouse) is used to help ease the baby's head out.

Jaundice—A common and usually harmless condition in newborn babies, characterized by yellowing of the skin and the whites of the eyes. In rare cases, jaundice can be a sign of an underlying health condition or can lead to brain damage.

Lactose—A sugar found in milk.

Linea nigra—A brownish line extending from the belly button down to below the panty line that appears in most women during pregnancy and remains for about a year after giving birth.

Listeriosis—A serious infection caused by the bacterium *Listeria monocytogenes*.

Melanin—A brown pigment produced by the skin.

Menstruation—The monthly shedding of the uterine lining; also known as a period.

Meta-analysis—A way of combining the results of lots of different studies to get a more accurate picture of the risks or benefits of a treatment.

MRI (magnetic resonance imaging)—A type of scan that uses strong magnets and radio waves to produce detailed images of the inside of the body.

National Health Service (NHS)—The UK's equivalent of the U.S.'s CDC.

National Institute for Health and Clinical Excellence (NICE)—The UK's organization that offers evidence-based guidance to doctors.

Neural tube defect—A birth defect of the brain and spinal cord.

Nipple confusion—When a baby develops a preference for feeding from a bottle rather than the breast.

Ovulation—The monthly release of a mature egg by the ovaries.

Oxytocin—A hormone involved in triggering labor and breast-feeding; also implicated in social bonding.

Peer review—A form of scientific self-regulation in which a study is critically read and reviewed by a researcher's peers before publication.

Pelvic-floor muscles—A group of muscles running between the pubic bone and tailbone that help support the bladder, vagina, uterus, and bowels.

Perineal tear—A tear to the perineum that often occurs during childbirth. Tears are classified into four categories, with a first-degree tear the most superficial and a fourth-degree tear being the most serious, extending into the anus and rectum.

Perineum—The area of tissue between the vagina and anus.

Placebo—An inactive substance or mock treatment often used as a control in clinical studies to compare the effectiveness of the real treatment.

Placenta—The organ that connects a developing baby to its mother's uterus and allows the exchange of oxygen, nutrients, and waste products between the two blood supplies.

Postnatal—The period of time after birth.

Preterm—The birth of a baby before thirty-seven weeks of pregnancy.

Progesterone—The pregnancy hormone that keeps the placenta working, keeps the lining of the uterus nice and thick, and stimulates breast growth.

Prolactin—The hormone that stimulates breast development and milk production.

Prostaglandins—Substances with many roles within the body, but which stimulate the cervix to soften and open, and the uterus to contract during birth.

Reflux—When the milk a baby has swallowed travels back up its food pipe and into its mouth.

Relaxin—Pregnancy hormone that causes the ligaments of the uterus and pelvis to loosen and relax to accommodate the growing baby.

REM sleep—A normal stage of sleep characterized by rapid movements of the eyes under the eyelids; also when dreaming is thought to occur.

Serotonin—Chemical that regulates mood, appetite, and sleep in the brain.

Sex ratio—The proportion of male to female births in a population.

Skin-to-skin contact—The practice of placing babies naked on their mothers' bare chests after birth.

Stages of labor—Labor is often divided into three stages: the first stage, when the uterus is contracting and the cervix opening; the second stage, when the baby is moving down the birth canal; and the third stage, when the placenta is delivered.

Sudden infant death syndrome (SIDS)—The sudden, unexpected, and unexplained death of an apparently healthy baby; also known as crib death.

Swaddling—The practice of wrapping babies in a blanket or cloth in order to restrict the movement of their limbs.

Syntocinon—A synthetic form of oxytocin sometimes given to kick-start or speed up labor.

Thyroid—A gland that produces a number of hormones controlling how quickly the body uses energy, makes proteins, and responds to other hormones.

Transcutaneous electrical nerve stimulation (TENS)—Involves the delivery of electrical impulses across the skin to block the transmission of pain signals.

Trimester—Pregnancy is often divided into three trimesters, with the first trimester marking weeks one to twelve of pregnancy; the second trimester marking weeks thirteen to twenty-eight; and the third trimester marking the final stage of pregnancy.

Ultrasound—A scan that uses sound waves to create images of the inside of the body.

Ventouse—A vacuum device that is applied to the baby's head to gently help pull it out of the mother's body.

Weaning—The introduction of solid foods to a baby's diet.

About the Author

Linda Geddes is a London-based journalist who writes about biology, medicine, and technology. Born in Cambridge, she graduated from Liverpool University with a first-class degree in cell biology. She has worked as both a news editor and reporter for *New Scientist* magazine, and has received numerous awards for her journalism, including the Association of British Science Writers' award for best investigative journalism. She is married with two young children, Matilda and Max.